HOWEVER WE CAN

A No-Shame Journey to Motherhood

Rena Ejiogu

Editorial Project Management: Karen Rowe, karen@karenrowe.com

Cover Design: Antonio Garcia, thisisagm.com

Author Image courtesy of Andrew Hite

Interior Layout: Ljiljana Pavkov

Printed in the United States of America

FIRST EDITION

Library of Congress

ISBN: 978-1-63649-885-0 (paperback)

ISBN: 978-1-63649-886-7 (eBook)

Published by

10 9 8 7 6 5 4 3 2 1

To Uche,
We got our family.

"We can do hard things—it's the impossible that takes a little longer."

— *Alan Packer*

TABLE OF

Contents

HOWEVER
WE CAN

A NOTE TO

Readers

THIS BOOK OUTLINES MY JOURNEY OF INFERTILITY. I TRIED every possible procedure and every possible solution—medical or otherwise—in my quest to become a mother. I used to be very tight-lipped about my journey; I didn't want to bother anyone with the details of the emotional roller coaster I was on. But as time went on, I got very lonely. I felt like no one understood.

After an eight-year stint in and out of clinics, seeing doctor after doctor, suffering loss after loss, I started talking about it. And you know what I found? I was not alone at all. In fact, there were a lot of friends and friends of friends who were experiencing some form of fertility issue. In a weird way, it was comforting to know I wasn't the only one. So, why the secrecy? Why are we groomed not to talk about certain things? I decided to try to stop that cycle and create a new trend—to speak up, speak loudly, speak proudly, and support one another.

When I felt an inner calling to help other women going through the fertility process, I had no idea what form that help would take. I considered many different online plat-forms—Instagram, blogs, podcasts. But anytime I would think about pursuing one of those paths, I would block myself with a wall of excuses as to why it wasn't possible. *I'm too busy; I don't know how; Would anyone even be interested?* The list went on.

But I kept coming back to my desire to help people. As our second child grew older, the pull inside me to share our story grew stronger. When I was mulling over how to bring my vision to life, a random post popped up on my Facebook feed offering support in writing a book. It felt right. I realized that if I didn't take that chance then, it was never going to happen.

I now know many women and couples dealing with similar heartbreak. Infertility can be very dark, emotional, and confusing. This book is designed to help those going through what, for us, can be one of the toughest obsta-cles in life...trying to have a baby.

My message to you is: You are not alone. My ride was rough and emotional—but I got through it, and you will, too...however you can. I learned through my journey to be open, honest, and to trust my intuition about what feels right for me. Our bodies will always guide us. By sharing our story, my ultimate goal is to create a safe zone, free of judgment and full of comfort, hope, knowledge, and so much love.

I know you may not be in the sharing phase yet, and that's okay. It took me a long time to get here and every-one's journey is different. But if you're reading this and it resonates just a little bit or gives you that glimmer of hope that you need, then writing this book was worth it.

CHAPTER ONE:

Our Love Story

My husband, Uche, and I went to the same high school. I was in grade ten and he was in grade twelve. We did not have the same circle of friends and we actually never spoke in school, but he was this hot basketball player—6'3" with broad shoulders, perfectly round biceps, thick black hair, and a wide bright smile—who I noticed and liked from afar.

I was at a basketball pep rally where our high school basketball team was playing our city's professional football league, believe it or not (some of the professional football players came to the school to play against the basketball team). I was sitting in the stands with my best friend, and Uche was on the court when all of a sudden, I screamed, "Dunk it again, Uche!" He looked at me, confused, but dunked the basketball. *He's in love with me*, I thought.

That was pretty much the extent of our high school relationship. Friends have told me that I would make them walk the long way to class so we could pass the gym to see if Uche was playing. I don't remember that, but I wouldn't put it past me. My mom remembers me talking about him and being opposed to me dating an older guy. Before long, he graduated. When I was in grade eleven, his sister came into grade ten, so I still felt a connection with him, although she and I never talked either.

Fast forward ten years: It was November 2007. I was twenty-six years old and had temporarily moved back to Calgary...or so I thought. I had gone to Ontario for university and ironically, so had Uche, although we attended different schools; he was at Ottawa University and I was at Wilfred Laurier University. One night, I was at a club with mutual friends that I did not know were mutual friends at the time. I saw Uche walk by and my stomach dropped. "Oh my God, that's Uche," I said, to no one in particular. His buddy, who was with me, asked me how I knew him. I told him we had gone to high school together. "Uche has a girlfriend," he said, to which I replied, "I never asked."

However, later in the night after having some liquid courage, I walked right up to Uche and said, "Hey, I don't know if you remember me. My name is Rena, we went to high school together. I used to have the biggest crush on you."

He gave me an up and down look and said, "Hey, you're my number one fan."

I laughed. "You remember that?"

"Nobody really has fans in high school," he gave me one of his wide, toothy smiles. We more or less left the conversation at that.

The next weekend was my staff Christmas party. A group of us from work decided we were going to go to that same club after the party. I dressed in my holiday best—a fitted black-and-white, short-sleeved, above-the-knee, satin, floral-printed dress that highlighted my slender, athletic build and black thigh- high stockings, to which I am thankful my friend introduced me. (I hate nylons and tights; these stockings were comfortable and sexy.) To finish the look, I wore knee-high, black leather, 2.5-inch stiletto boots, bringing my height up to nearly six feet. I had straightened my thick brown curly hair that night, something which I rarely do, but it felt great, bobbing and swaying just above my shoulders.

While standing at the bar with my friend, I kept getting pushed. The place was packed. At one point, I got pushed so hard that I turned around to yell at the insensitive jerk who was shoving me. It was Uche.

I looked up at him—he now stood only three inches taller than me—and he looked down at me. "Oh, hi again." The irritation I felt melted away as I flashed him one of my thin-lipped, dimpled smiles. We started talking. My friend wanted to leave but she could tell I was having a good time, so she went up to Uche and said, "Look, I have to go, but you're a really nice guy, so if I leave Rena here…"

"Don't worry. I got her," Uche finished for her.

That night he asked me for my phone number.

"No, because I hear you have a girlfriend," I said.

"What? Where did you hear that? And not anymore. We broke up and she is moving out."

"Well, I don't want to get involved in that situation," I replied. To my knowledge, I did not give him my number. But early the next morning, he called me.

"How did you get my number?" I asked.

"You don't remember?" No. I didn't remember. "Before you left, you wrote your number down and put it in my pocket and said, "Shh, don't tell anyone." Again, liquid courage.

"Oh, that was a good move," I said, surprised. And we have been talking ever since.

● ● ●

I have always known that I wanted to be a mom. Before I was even a teenager, I loved kids. I started babysitting as soon as I was old enough, would play with my friends' younger siblings whenever I could, and was always the first in line to volunteer to mentor the little ones at school. When I was at synagogue and was bored with the service, I would sit outside in the main area with the little kids, babysitting whoever was there. I was drawn to kids and they were drawn to me. I loved their innocence, their imagination. We would sing songs, play hide-and-seek, and do whatever we could do quietly while our parents were in the sanctuary. My parents have a picture of me sitting outside the sanctuary with a group of five kids around me and a little one on my lap. It was my happy place.

So, when the topic of children came up on my first date with Uche in February 2008, I didn't flinch. We went to a lounge for drinks and were sitting in a quiet booth when he casually asked, "Do you want kids?" It was a loaded question for so early in the relationship, but I didn't hesitate.

"Yes, absolutely."

"How many do you want?" he persisted.

"I don't know, two or three. How many do you want?"

He smiled, with no hint of sarcasm in his voice, and said, "Thirteen."

A "normal" person may have spit out her drink with such a response, but not me. "Oh, okay. Maybe we can talk," I replied, just as casually. He later told me that, because I didn't freak out or run off, he knew right then, *This is the girl I'm going to marry.* He was joking; he didn't want thirteen kids. But he also knew he really wanted kids.

For my part, I knew instantly that he was like no other guy I'd ever dated. I very much had a type; I had previously dated guys who tended to be jerks, players, or those who would cheat on me. Uche, on the other hand, was very kind, polite, and super smart. He was working for an oil and gas company as a reservoir technologist. Of course, he didn't look bad either—I remembered him as a jock, but in his freshly pressed blazer, he sure did clean up nice. Conversation flew effortlessly and we laughed together readily.

We went on a few more dates, but our relationship moved very slowly (also very different from previous relationships I'd had). Roughly six weeks after our first date, I made the decision that I was going to buy a house and move to Ontario, which was over 2,000 miles away. I was working for my dad as a dental hygienist at the time. I loved working for him; I loved his office, I loved my colleagues, I loved my patients, and I was excelling in my career. Hygiene is one of those careers you can do anywhere, but once you get in a good office, you want to stay there. What drew me to Ontario was that my sister was there, along with my niece and nephew, who were growing so quickly. They were already one and three years old, and I wanted to be close to them. Despite my high standards for employers, I decided to work with a temporary staffing agency in Ontario and made the move in April, 2008.

Why was I so willing to leave Uche behind? He was, after all, the only boyfriend my family had ever approved of. The truth is, I really wanted him to tell me to stay before I went to Ontario, but he didn't. And so, I moved. I was in my new house for a week when Uche showed up at my doorstep and said, "You're it for me. I don't want to date anyone else. I love you."

I quietly and politely replied, "Thanks!" At that moment, everything felt like it was moving so fast. I knew that Uche was the type of guy who wouldn't just say "I love you" to anyone; I needed to make sure I loved him too before I just blurted it back. But once he said it, I started taking down the wall of protection I had built due to past relationships and realized that I loved him, too. He had only come to spend the weekend with me, but he kept postponing his flight and ended up staying for a week. By the end of May, we drove back to Calgary together and moved in together right away.

Trying Naturally

From the start, we worked well together. We were still in our twenties, so we had a carefree, fun, easy-going life-style. We would go to the mountains, go skiing, and go floating down the river near where we were living. On weekends we would meet up with friends at bars or go to dinner parties. At the same time, we were "adulting"; we bought a house together in July, moved into it in August, and by February 2009, he proposed. This time, it was an easy decision to make. We knew we were meant to be together.

We stopped using protection a couple of months before our August 2009 wedding. We thought, *Whatever happens, will happen.* When I first started trying to conceive, I had an idyllic vision of what would happen. I thought it was going to be easy because everybody around me was pregnant or getting pregnant and having no problems (or not talking about it if they were).

Growing up, my cycle was all over the place. To me, that was normal. I had never really had a regular window; it varied between a twenty-eight-day cycle, thirty-five-day cycle, or a thirty-eight-day cycle, and sometimes it wouldn't come at all. It had been like that my whole life, and I never had a doctor tell me I might have difficulty getting pregnant. It didn't even cross my mind that I would ever have difficulty conceiving.

I didn't know anything about cycle monitoring until we dove into trying to have kids. Learning how to chart my cycle was not one of those things I'd sat down with my parents to talk about as a young girl, or ever learned in school. As the months went on and we weren't getting pregnant, I started to research the topic of fertility, trying any advice anyone offered about what worked for them. I'm not really a reader, but someone recommended the book *Taking Charge of Your Fertility*, by Toni Weschler. That's when I discovered there is only a seventy-two-hour window per cycle when a woman can actually get pregnant. I followed the charts in the book about how to monitor my cycle and know my absolute optimal, most fertile time. Every morning, I did a temperature check and cervical mucus check, following the author's protocol exactly. I charted my results, which looked like a line graph.

I ended up seeking the help of a naturopathic doctor because my charts didn't make sense to me. There should have been a certain point in the graph where everything lined up, which would be my most fertile time, but nothing lined up for me the way it should have; my temperature would never match my mucus, which would never match the position of my cervix. It was frustrating and confusing. As it turned out, we had been following a schedule that never worked for me because my cycles were so long that day fourteen wasn't my ovulation day (the typical ovulation day for someone with a regular, twenty-eight-day cycle). In addition, my ovulation days were different every month because my cycle lengths were different.

We started looking into alternative medicine. I did acupuncture. My naturopathic doctor put me on fish oil supplements. She had me on an HMF neuro probiotic and a pH balancer. All of these were supposed to help make the environment inside me the best it could be for conception.

Uche and I started having sex every other day, from days ten to twenty of my cycle, hoping to hit the jackpot that way. The love was gone, I'll just put it that way. We had to do it because we wanted something, not because we wanted each other. Physical intimacy became so robotic. There were some days when we really did not want to have sex, but we forced ourselves to because that's what we were told to do. Uche felt the same—it was a chore. There was no sensuality, no flirtation, no foreplay, no mental connection—just a lot of pressure. We did manage to maintain intimacy in other ways. We would go on dates to emotionally connect, and resort to other types of physical intimacy. I joked that it felt like we were in junior high.

Of course, everyone had advice for us. People recommended various solutions:

"If you prop yourself up on a pillow, that helps things go in and stay in more."

"If you ride like you're on a bicycle, upside down and backward, that works."

"If you do a headstand, you're more likely to get pregnant."

"If you eat this hideous food, it increases your chances of conceiving."

We heard...and implemented...all these ridiculous things in the name of fertility. I did them all, and none of them worked for me—or so I thought.

I didn't realize it then, but during that time, I did get pregnant. Uche and I were out for a walk in the neighborhood one day when all of a sudden, I had such immense pain that I had to sit down on the side of the road as cars were driving by us. Once I was able to get up, we walked home and I went to the bathroom and saw a ton of blood and a little bean about an inch long; I just thought it was tissue from a heavy period. Now I know it was a miscarriage.

CHAPTER TWO:

Fertility Clinics

THE STANDARD PROCEDURE FOR TREATING INFERTILITY IS TO try naturally for a year before going to a fertility clinic. After a year of trying to get pregnant naturally and being unsuccessful, a patient of mine got us into the Regional Fertility Clinic in Calgary, which had an extremely long waitlist. At the time, it was the only fertility clinic in southern Alberta; it was associated with one of the main hospitals in the city, so it was very busy.

My initial consult was July 16, 2010. Uche and I went to the appointment together, parking outside the brown brick building that looked straight out of the 1980s. The similarities to an older era didn't stop there. As we entered the second-floor office, we were met by a receptionist who seemed to be on autopilot. She immediately handed us papers to sign without saying much; it was not a very personable experience from the start. She was very short with answers to our questions, steering us towards the waiting room which was set up in a modular formation with chairs aligned in rows. It was packed with people across all demographics. There was a stack of reading material and an area in the corner with a few kids' toys. From there, we could hear the phone at the reception desk going unanswered.

"It feels a bit disorganized, don't you think?" I whispered to Uche. He nodded. Our gut feeling was that this wasn't a clinic we would feel comfortable in, but we tried to set that feeling aside. We were so grateful to have gotten the appointment and tried our best to maintain our high hopes and positive expectations. Before long, we were called into a small corner consultation room with a round table and chairs. The walls were drab white with nothing on them; it felt cold and unwelcoming. Despite appearances, we were looking forward to meeting the head doctor, who we had been told we were lucky to be assigned to.

Uche and I sat on one side of the table, closest to the door, and waited for the doctor to arrive.

"Rena," he walked in and acknowledged me, but not Uche. From the start, it felt wrong. The doctor had long, stringy gray hair and seemingly no personality. He took no time to make small talk or establish rapport and instead took a seat across from us and started his line of questioning.

"What are your medical histories?"

"How long have you been trying to get pregnant?"

"Have you ever been pregnant before?"

"Has your husband gotten anyone pregnant before?"

"Do you have a family history of infertility?"

He took notes, without looking up, as I answered his questions. It felt like he was going through the motions. We were just another block on the conveyor belt. The doctor then explained what the protocol was moving forward, starting with all the testing we would need to get done as a preliminary assessment.

For any woman who wants to get pregnant and can't, impatience is palpable. It always feels like nothing is happening fast enough and everything needs to get done yesterday. Getting the appointment at the clinic had felt like a big step forward—but once I was there, I wasn't sure what we had gotten into.

The doctor, for whatever reason, didn't take the time to learn Uche's name, which really bothered me. In a situation like this, people need extra love and we just didn't feel it. Also, whenever the doctor would talk to us, he would never look at Uche. Even if Uche was talking to him, he'd look up at the ceiling.

We wondered if we should have trusted our gut feelings enough to leave the clinic. However, it was also the only clinic available in our city. We did what we thought we had to do. So, we stayed. Overall, I left the appointment feeling dissatisfied, unimportant, like I was just a number, and yet I was also eager to start the process.

Fertility Testing

After the first consult at the Calgary Clinic, testing was done to check if there were any fertility issues with either of us. Uche got a sperm analysis to test motility and make sure his swimmers were swimming straight rather than in circles. It was not a sexy process. He had to go into a private room, stacked with trashy adult magazines that were old and well-used, alongside a TV with an outdated program running to help with "stimulation" — which he shared were not much help! After doing his business in a cup, he slid it through a window that connects to the lab. He also had to have full bloodwork done, as well as an STD screening.

As for me, I had an HSG (hysterosalpingography) test. They injected dye into me using a thin catheter through my cervix, and watched via x-ray to see if the dye went through my uterus and my fallopian tubes properly. The exam was to check if there were any blockages or if everything flowed properly. I was excited because we were at that next step; I was also nervous because I was hoping nothing was wrong. I remember thinking, *What are they going to find?*

I grew up in a medical family, but I'd never had something like that done before. I could watch the whole thing on the screen, so it was kind of neat to see the dye go through my body. I experienced some light cramping, but it wasn't overly uncomfortable or invasive. Once I saw the dye go through, it offered a bit of relief because I knew that my tubes were functioning properly. I got the results right away. The doctor confirmed that everything was looking good and the results were clear. *Okay, check that step off the list*, I thought.

I also had hormone testing through bloodwork (again, full work up for basic virology, STD screening, blood type, and rubella). I went back for bloodwork a couple of times, depending on the day of my cycle, so they could monitor my hormone levels (follicle-stimulating hormone, or FSH, and estrogen). Finally, I had to have an ultrasound done to check my uterus, ovarian reserve, and antral follicle count (AFC).

The outcome of all that testing was normal—everything was functioning and working as it was supposed to. There was no medical reason they could find as to why we weren't conceiving naturally. They called it "unexplained infertility," which is very broad and annoying. I almost wanted them to find something; if everything was functioning normally, why weren't we pregnant? If we don't know the source of the problem, it's hard to fix.

Clomid

We met with the doctor again, who outlined the whole scenario for us moving forward. "Start with Clomid®," he said. "If that doesn't work, then move to an IUI. If that doesn't work, then try in vitro fertilization (IVF)...;" he continued listing the step-by-step process without giving much explanation, which caused us to reiterate our initial feeling of the operation being run like a conveyor belt; care was not personalized. As the doctor was going through the list with us, I *never* thought we would make it down the whole production line, and beyond! I was super hopeful at that point, and so was Uche. He actually didn't think we needed to do any of this at all—that we'd get pregnant naturally with time.

Clomid is recommended after trying naturally for a year and not conceiving. It's a medication to make a woman ovulate more than one egg and increase her chances of getting pregnant. At our second consult on September 3, 2010, we received my prescription for

Clomid, which I took for three months on days three to seven of my cycle. Despite being on Clomid, we were still trying naturally to get pregnant, but to no avail.

IUI

After trying naturally, taking all the tests, taking Clomid, and still not getting pregnant, the next step is Intrauterine Insemination (IUI), which is unprofessionally known as "turkey basting." It is a type of artificial insemination, where sperm that have been washed and concentrated are placed directly in the uterus around the time the ovary releases one or more eggs to be fertilized.

We had an IUI on January 17, 2011, February 14, 2011, and March 19, 2011. At this point, I was still on Clomid, which I ended up taking for a total of six months—which some doctors say is the maximum time to be on that drug. During this process, I had to call the clinic (the "period hotline") on day one of my cycle and leave a message. Then, a nurse would call me back with instructions on when to start each medication and when to begin cycle monitoring. I monitored my cycle using an ovulation predictor kit. When 'the time was right,' I called the nurse back and the clinic chose the best day for the procedure to have the highest chance of success.

"If you don't get pregnant within those five months, chances are it's not going to work for you and it's time to move onto your next step," the doctor told us. By March, I still wasn't pregnant. At that point, the doctor called us in and decided he wanted to do exploratory surgery on me to see if I had endometriosis or any sort of underlying condition.

There are four indicators of endometriosis—long or irregular cycles/excessive bleeding, infertility, pain during intercourse, and painful cramps. I only had two of the four—painful cramps and irregular periods. (And now, I realize, infertility.) Uche got really frustrated and told the doctor, "You're not cutting my wife open just to see if she has something." The doctor said, "If I do see something, I'll repair it then." It made no sense to us to have that procedure, so we finally left that clinic and got a second opinion at a fertility clinic in Burlington, Ontario called ONE Fertility.

Finding Our Place

We went all the way to Ontario from Alberta because my sister Jana and her husband Matt were there. Being able to stay with them took some stress off. I had asked my sister, who was a NICU nurse at the time, for recommendations and this clinic had great reviews.

At the Alberta clinic, I felt very rushed, like I was a number; it was not patient-centered care. The Ontario clinic was run very differently. It was a smaller clinic, with only one floor. As I entered the double glass doors, my eyes landed on a coffee/tea/hot chocolate station. *That's sweet*, I thought. The waiting room was a big, bright open area with comfy chairs lined up in rows—the good kind, with wooden frames, not the cheapy plastic ones. There was also a big-screen TV mounted on the wall.

The front desk had a couple of women working at it, both of whom smiled and greeted us as we walked in. *This place feels friendly*, I thought. The color scheme of

the clinic was a warm burgundy-and-neutral combina-
tion. It was very soothing and comforting. I relaxed a little.
After checking in, we took our seats in the waiting room.
I was pleasantly surprised that they carried some of my
favorite magazines. *Great, I can catch up on my celebrity
gossip!* Our wait time was minimal.

When our names were called, we were greeted by a
nurse who took us to the consultation room. The first
thing she did was ask how to pronounce Uche's name
and our last name. She practiced it with our guidance,
making sure she knew how to say it properly. (There was
never an issue with Uche's name at this clinic. Everyone
knew it, and called him by it with ease.) She, too, smiled
brightly and asked us questions about how we were. It
felt genuine, like we were already friends.

Again, we didn't wait long before the doctor came
in smiling, as if we had known each other for years. She
shook our hands and said *both* of our names, which was
surprising and a relief. She sat at her desk and asked us
to go over our history—where we were in treatment, and
what brought us in to see her. I think I did all the talking,
or most of it! Once I was done, she grabbed my arm,
looked me straight in the eyes, and said, "I'm sorry you're
going through this. I'm here for you."

I instantly started crying. It felt good; it felt right. This
was the first doctor who showed genuine caring. There
was compassion, empathy, and personal-based care.
We had only gone in for a second opinion but fell in love
with the clinic's style, the treatments, and the staff's open
arms, so we decided to stay. Finding a doctor that made
me feel that way was everything in this process.

CHAPTER THREE:

IVF

When it comes to IUIs, three is the magic number. My doctor at the Ontario clinic reaffirmed that it was time for me to move on to IVF. "Look," she told us, "we could do another IUI, but if you've had three with no success, chances are it's not going to work. I would hate for you to spend more money on IUIs and then have to end up needing IVF anyway." We thought, *Well, we might as well go the IVF route. It will give us a better chance.*

Never in a million years had I thought we'd need to go that route. I never pictured needing help from doctors and science to have a baby. Maybe it was a subconscious defense because IVF has such a heaviness to it, but my belief that we would conceive naturally was reinforced by being told by every doctor we saw that we were both functional—"unexplained infertility" meant there was no known problem.

IVF is also expensive, and that was really scary. For people who do not like to spend money, this was a big chunk of our savings. But to us, it was necessary. We were determined to have a baby. The process itself was also scary because it was unknown. Not many people talk about the process, so the energy behind "IVF"—at least to me—was that it was serious. I thought, *Really, this is what we have to do!*

To undergo IVF, both Uche and I had to go through a mandatory program where the entire process is explained, because it's very intense. Typically, we'd both have to be there in person, but because I was in Ontario and Uche was still in Calgary, they made an exception for us and I was able to attend the meeting with Uche on a FaceTime call.

I sat at the very front of the class so that I could hold my phone up and make sure that he could see and hear the instructor, who explained in detail everything the process could involve. He went over the medications we would be on and why we'd be on them, the different grades of embryos—showing us microscopic pictures of what a healthy embryo that would be perfect for transfer would look like—and the costs of each procedure. Of course, every case would be unique and not everyone would need every step of the procedure, but we learned about them all.

It was a lot to take in, and I found myself wishing Uche were there with me in person; just being able to hold his hand would have helped. Without him there for emotional support, I treated the seminar more like a university class; I tried to take myself out of it emotionally to get through. I focused on taking notes and recording the facts.

Medications and Egg Retrieval

I started my medications for IVF on January 3, 2012, which included three injections daily for five days. I could choose whether to inject myself in the stomach or my thigh. I chose my thigh because the thought of stabbing myself in the stomach just did not appeal.

Gonal-F® and Luveris® are follicle (egg) stimulating hormones, used to stimulate an egg to develop and mature. The other medication, Suprefact®, prevents ovulation. All of these injections and medications are taken to produce as many eggs as possible; they swell the ovaries.

I had my sister give me my injections the first time. The next time, she was at work so I called a friend of mine who works in insurance; she gave me my injection because I just couldn't do it. Finally, there was a time when neither my sister nor my friend was available, so I had no choice.

All right, I guess I've got to do this, I thought.

I sat down at the kitchen table. I had laid out all my supplies and medications neatly in front of me. I marked the dosage on the Gonal-F by turning the end of the pen until the right dosage appeared in the little window on the side. I then filled a syringe with Luveris from the vial, making sure there were no air bubbles in the syringe. I stared at the shots in front of me for a bit, summoning the courage.

I grabbed Gonal-F first. It was a smaller needle. I took hold of my right upper thigh with my left hand, the injection pen in my right hand. The voice in my head was strongly giving me a pep talk, *You can totally do this! How hard can it be?* Then I closed my eyes and inserted the needle.

Wait, that's it? That was so not a big deal! Then came the Luveris...that one had a bigger needle and more medication. Still, I managed to insert the needle.

It burned and didn't feel great in comparison to the first injection, but it was still not worth the panic I was in beforehand. From then on, I gave myself my shots wherever, whenever, without even thinking twice. It got to the point where I did it so much, I could do it in the dark. I had red dots down both sides of my thighs because I would alternate them, so I didn't wear a bathing suit for a while.

By the end of those five days, I felt very sore and bloated. I had to walk very carefully. There were rules I had to follow—you can't lift, you can't twist, you can't make sudden movements because you run the risk of your ovary collapsing and twisting (they are really heavy because you are producing so many eggs).

On January 7, the fifth and final day, I was instructed to take the Gonal-F injection plus an additional medication called Ovidrel®, which would make me ovulate, or release my eggs. Then on January 9, I went in for egg retrieval. For this, I was under conscious sedation; the way the doctor described it was that it's like drinking a whole bottle of wine. You know what's going on, but you don't really care. After the fact, I had pain on my left side, but nothing I couldn't handle.

I was lying on a bed, as if I were getting a Pap smear, with my legs strapped. There was a window that opened to the lab; modesty goes out the door in this situation. They showed the process on the ultrasound; it looked like a needle going in but it's more like a scoop. They retrieved as many eggs as they could. Uche was with me for the egg retrieval, although not in the room itself during the procedure. Not only was it comforting having him nearby, but the nurses and the whole staff were wonderful. My doctor was with me to talk through the procedure; we were even joking around. At this stage, I was still feeling hopeful and excited. *This is my next step and it is going to work* was my prevailing attitude.

I am thankful I responded quite well, and we ended up retrieving nine eggs. I was given a choice once my eggs were retrieved. For lack of a better explanation, picture a Petri dish with your egg in it. You can either put the sperm sample in with the egg and hope the sperm finds the egg or do something called intracytoplasmic sperm injection (ICSI), where they inseminate the egg with the sperm. We decided to do the ICSI because of course, it would increase our chances of conception.

Through ICSI, seven of our eggs were fertilized, so we were down two. The doctors determine which embryos are sufficient or "good" based on a grading system. If you picture a pizza, the embryos have to have a certain thickness around them—sort of like the crust on the pizza. They also have to look symmetrical, like a pizza slice. They use the eggs' grade to determine which ones will be implanted. If the egg is a lower grade, they won't even use the embryo.

This office was great because they will never implant more than two eggs in a patient—the maximum they will do is twins. There are regulations in Canada to prevent an "Octomom" scenario, and some clinics have their own limitation policies as well. The doctor told us that we had a really good chance at conceiving, because of my age and because of the quality of our embryos, and that we could even have twins.

Embryo Transfer and Waiting for a Positive Test

On January 12, I did a fresh embryo cycle transfer. The remaining embryos were frozen so they would be useable in the future. If a frozen embryo transfer cycle is performed, those embryos have to go through a thawing process, and some do not survive. The chances of getting pregnant are higher with a fresh cycle than with a frozen cycle.

Uche and I were taken into a small, quiet room with the lights dimmed low.

"Please confirm your name and birthday," the nurse said to me. I had to say it out loud and look at it printed on the sample. Once we confirmed we were the owners of the sample, the procedure started.

I laid back on the table. Uche held my hand. The atmosphere was relaxing and pleasant. A lab technician transferred the eggs to the doctor through a window for the doctor to implant using ultrasound imaging. Two of the fertilized embryos were loaded into a catheter, then inserted through my cervix and into my uterus. I could see the embryos being inserted on the ultrasound, which was pretty exciting. When they let go of the embryos, they floated around in my uterus looking for a spot to implant. As they floated, they were lit up with a flash of light that only lasted for a moment; they took a picture of that flash and gave it to me—my first ultrasound pic! We were feeling optimistic and hopeful; after all, we *saw* the embryos go in.

After the first transfer, I left my sister's place in Ontario and went back home to Calgary. I was put on

Endometrin® (progesterone) via vaginal suppository to help make things move along. I was also told to limit physical activity.

After having an embryo transfer, there is a two-week waiting period before finding out if it worked. Those two weeks are...how can I describe it? Agonizing! I tried to go about my life as normally as I possibly could. I went back to work, working part-time at the dental office, which was a healthy distraction from sitting and worrying. If my mind wasn't on a task, then anxious thoughts would flood in.

I was still feeling hopeful and excited, but I was also really nervous. I wanted it to work so badly, and yet I also wanted to relax in order to make sure the environment within me was good for conception. I limited my social activity, didn't drink alcohol, ate healthy food, and min- imized my exercise. I was essentially acting as if I were already pregnant, to give the process the best possible outcome. I was also conscious of having just spent a ton of money on the procedure. I wasn't about to risk losing our investment.

I was trying to be in tune with what I was feeling and took anything out of the ordinary as a sign of possible pregnancy, which took a lot out of me early on. Even when I was trying not to think about it, somewhere in my head, I was thinking about it. I never really had a problem sleeping, but every time I woke up, I would be conscious of the fact that I was trying to get pregnant. *I'm one day closer*, I told myself every day. There was nothing I could do but wait.

Finally, it was time to take a pregnancy test. Normally this would be done at the clinic using bloodwork, but because I was back in Calgary, I took a urine test at home. And...it came back positive! I was so excited! I called Uche at work to let him know the news. We were ecstatic! Then I called the clinic in Ontario. "Guess what? It worked!" I told my nurse.

But a couple of days later, I started bleeding. I didn't have any pain; it just seemed like a period, but I was devastated. Uche was at work, and I felt so alone. I sat on our bed, reached for my phone, and called the clinic. Immediately, I started bawling.

"We're so sorry, but sometimes this happens," the nurse told me. "Because we didn't do the test via bloodwork, which checks your hormone levels for pregnancy, you could have gotten a false positive." Or, I could have miscarried, which was devastating to consider. In my head, IVF was supposed to be a sure shot, and it wasn't. I felt defeated. Those were two losses, right there.

I started questioning everything I did and wondered why it wasn't working. *Is there anything I could have done differently?!* The questioning was torture. Whether trying to get pregnant naturally or using science to get pregnant, there are a ton of extra hormones going through the body that cause very high and very low mood swings in an instant. The trigger for me was seeing any type of blood; blood would put me into an instant panic.

To see a positive test and then not be pregnant chipped away at my hope. I started to prepare myself for disappointment and to talk about what we would do if it didn't work. Before IVF, I would never even allow myself to think, *if it doesn't work*. I was adamant. *I'm going to make this happen. I'm going to do whatever it takes*, I thought.

Life seemed to go on as usual on the outside; nobody knew what we were going through aside from a few select friends and our families—and even they only knew we were having trouble getting pregnant. Meanwhile, our friends started getting pregnant. We were happy for them, but so frustrated and discouraged that it wasn't happening for us. Those that knew that we were trying would say, "It's going to be okay, just relax."

There is a funny meme going around that says, "Never in the history of calming down has anyone ever calmed down by being told to calm down." An article in the *Wall Street Journal* says "instructing people to calm down typically has the reverse effect." When I was tracking my cycle and also being told to relax and calm my body, it was very hard to do—especially when everything was so scheduled and rigid. I had to investigate every inch of my body to "make a miracle" happen. When people told me to relax, I wanted to give them the big middle finger.

Despite having Uche as my rock, it was a very lonely time. Because nobody really talks about their experiences, I'd been groomed not to, as well. "Don't tell anyone you're doing IVF"; "Don't tell anyone you're pregnant until you're three months along"; "Don't tell anyone you're doing this because there's a stigma"; "If you open up about trying to get pregnant, it won't happen." The messaging is relentless.

We decided to keep trying; we still had five embryos left. I was put on two milligrams of Estrace® (similar to estrogen) taken orally twice daily. Then I went to Ontario and stayed with Jana and Matt again. On April 20, we did a frozen embryo transfer. This time, Uche had to stay in Calgary so Jana came with me for moral support.

It felt like having kids in daycare; the morning of the thawing process, they'd call me and give me a play-by-play update of our little embryos. "Okay, we've got your two embryos. We are going to start thawing them now." Then they'd call and let me know the progression of the thaw. Thankfully, both of our embryos did survive the thaw.

The doctor had a fun relationship with my sister; she would never use Jana's name, but would smile and address her, "Hi sister!" We were all laughing and in good spirits. We implanted two more embryos. As we looked at the ultrasound screen, we saw the flickers of light from the embryos as they passed into my uterus. This time only one of them floated around. The other one shot straight, with intent, to my uterine lining.

"Well, that one definitely stuck!" my sister commented. I looked at the doctor and the expression on her face confirmed she felt the same as Jana.

"Yes, that one shot out quick!" *Did it stick? Was it really going to work this time?* I knew what I saw, and I knew that they saw. I was extremely hopeful and excited, but also subconsciously prepared for the worst. As we drove back to my sister's house, we chatted about the transfer, and Jana was convinced.

She said it again, "That one totally stuck! I'd put money on it!"

CHAPTER FOUR:

Pregnancy and Delivery

SINCE THERE IS A TWO-WEEK WAITING PERIOD AFTER IMPLAN-tation, and because I miscarried during the first round of IVF, I'd already decided that I was going to stay at Jana and Matt's house near the clinic for those two weeks. During that time, we had to give my young niece and nephew some rules. They were not allowed to jump on Auntie, nor touch her stomach. Jana, being a nurse, was very good at explaining why to them.

As the days progressed, I became more and more excited, because I was closer to the day of the pregnancy test and hadn't had any more bleeding incidents. I was also apprehensive and mentally preparing myself for a fall by not letting myself get *too* excited.

One night in particular, Jana and Matt went out and I was home babysitting my niece and nephew. We had eaten tortellini, and just as Jana and Matt got home and walked through the door, I looked at them and got a whiff of something and felt sick. I ran to the kitchen sink, dry heaving. Jana and Matt started laughing.

"What's so funny?" I looked at them, incredulously. "Clearly, I'm not feeling well."

Matt said, "You're so pregnant right now."

"I don't know about that..." I said.

"Trust me, I have seen your sister pregnant twice. You are pregnant."

Ooh, maybe I am pregnant, I thought. I'd never had a smell make me feel so sick.

My parents flew in for the weekend to visit us all, but also because it was my birthday. The end of the two-week wait to find out if I was pregnant landed on my thirty-first birthday! When the waiting time was up, I went in for bloodwork in the morning with a hopeful heart. "I'll call you with the results in the afternoon," the nurse said, smiling. I couldn't wait.

A few hours later, I could hardly answer my phone fast enough.

"Hello?"

"Rena? This is the clinic. We have good news."

Ohmigod. "The test result came back positive." *Best birthday present EVER!*

I could barely contain my excitement. I wanted to cry and scream at the same time. I wanted so badly for Uche to be there. I called him right away to fill him in on the good news.

"Babe, guess what?" My voice said it all.

"No, really? We're pregnant?"

"Yes!" We cried tears of joy. We were beyond thrilled. But underneath there was still apprehension. We had experienced all those happy feelings the previous month when I'd gotten the positive urine test result, but then I started bleeding a few days later. We were understandably nervous. Still, this time felt different. I couldn't explain why, but it felt real.

I ran upstairs to tell everyone. "Guys! You were right! I can't believe it!"

"I knew it!" Matt said proudly.

My parents were thrilled for us as well. We were out to lunch together a couple of days later, still glowing from the news, when I had to use the bathroom. I had not expected to see what I did.

Noooo, this isn't happening! I couldn't believe it. I was bleeding...again. Already. Any type or amount of bleeding was a bad sign to me. It could be a clot. It could be a regular period. It could be a miscarriage. I came back out and looked at my mom. One glance, and she knew something was up. She followed me back to the bathroom and I started crying. I told her I was bleeding and right away she said, "We're going to the clinic." I wanted to call first and she said, "No, we're going." My parents drove me to the clinic; they did bloodwork and checked my hormone levels.

"We have good news and bad news," the nurse told me. "Bad news is you miscarried one embryo. Good news is, the other one stuck."

"Huh?" I said. Despite all the training we'd had about the process, I didn't even know you could miscarry one and keep one. I started to feel hopeful again. *I'm still pregnant!*

I felt relief as well as caution. I was so relieved that the IVF had worked and that things were progressing normally, but of course I had to be cautious because of my history. I didn't want to cause any issues.

I went back to Calgary and took off work through my first trimester. When I went back to work at twelve weeks, the excitement hit. My close work friends knew a bit about what we were going through and that I'd had some miscarriages. When I slowly started telling patients, it started to feel more real.

I went shopping with my mom, and she bought me some maternity clothes and baby clothes. She hated that we weren't finding out the gender because she wanted to do way more shopping than she felt she could. My mom and dad also gifted us big-ticket items, like a City Select stroller, which was so exciting. When we were closer to the due date, Uche's parents took us on a shopping spree to Babies 'R' Us to get us the essentials: burp cloths, a bathtub, baby washcloths, and lotions. I remember it felt like being on a game show; we had a shopping cart and I could put whatever I wanted in it. This was to be Uche's parents' first grandchild, so they were extremely excited to be able to participate.

I welcomed every single pregnancy symptom I had because it had been so difficult for us to conceive. If I wasn't feeling good, I embraced it. In terms of standard pregnancy side-effects, I was a bloodhound. I could smell everything. Smells would make me nauseous, but if I steered clear of what I didn't like, I was fine. I hated opening the fridge because the smell bothered me. I couldn't cook meat—anything meat-related grossed me out. I never had morning sickness or threw up, but sometimes I would gag while I ate. At the end of the afternoon, I would have low energy; I slept a lot. Every day Uche would get home from work and find me passed out on the couch in my scrubs. He'd make dinner and wake me up to eat and then I would go back to bed.

One of the greatest things I remember is that every day Uche would come home from work and rub my belly. He was constantly snuggling with our baby-to-be. Anytime the baby would kick, I'd grab Uche right away. He created a playlist and put his phone on my belly for the baby to listen to. Whenever a Frank Ocean song would come on, the baby would kick so hard that the phone would either fall off my belly or shake in tune with the beats.

We were learning about the female body, getting in tune with it, and paying attention to the physical changes that come along with pregnancy, i.e., food cravings or aversions, increased sense of smell, feeling baby flutters and movements, feeling muscles stretch as the baby grows, and bigger boobs—my favorite part! For example, during my first trimester, one of the only things that didn't make me feel sick was a certain brand of microwaveable macaroni, which is as disgusting as it sounds. I don't ordinarily eat processed food so Uche thought it must be good if I was eating it. We bought it by the freezer full, and one day Uche decided to eat some. My husband is not picky when it comes to food. I have only ever seen him not eat a meal once. He took one bite of the microwaveable macaroni and said, "This is trash. How are you eating this?" He couldn't eat it. A couple of weeks later, my love for the macaroni went away and I realized how nasty it was and stopped eating it. But I thank that microwaveable macaroni for getting me through my first trimester.

One night, Uche and I were watching a movie while lying on the couch. The baby turned, making it look like there was an alien in my stomach. Both Uche and I were grossed out but equally intrigued and amazed. I said, "Whoa. I had a big butt just sticking out of my stomach!" We walked through the pregnancy with a lot of curiosity, a lot of learning, and so much love. We were so relieved to be pregnant.

Ready to Deliver

Uche and I were extremely grateful that everything progressed normally and there were no concerns or complications. I was coasting through pregnancy. *Finally, something is going right!* I thought.

Right around this time, the *Twilight* novel series was very popular, and the movies were coming out. I liked to describe myself pregnant as turning into Bella Swan when she was changing into a vampire; when she is converted, she turns into this perfectly porcelain-skinned, beautiful, glowing figure with magical flowing hair. That's what I felt like. I never had any acne. My nails grew and were the best they've ever been. My hair, which is normally thick and coarse, was so soft and luscious and growing long. My skin was silky. However, toward the end of my pregnancy, I was so big. I gained forty pounds and it was all belly.

About a month or so before my due date, someone told me to put a garbage bag on top of the mattress cover so that if my water broke in bed, it wouldn't ruin the mattress. I thought that was such a good idea and did just that—oh, the things we learn! One night, Uche had gone out with a buddy to a local pub, which for some reason made me cranky. I was hormonal and feeling sad about missing out. He got to go out and here I was, big as a horse and crabby for no reason. Around 9 p.m., I went to bed. For some reason, although I hadn't checked it in weeks, I decided to check the garbage bag to make sure it was laid down properly. I hadn't yet fallen asleep when, within twenty minutes, I stood up wondering if I had just peed myself. I went to the bathroom dripping liquid down my legs, along with some clumpy white stuff. *This is weird*, I thought.

I went back to bed and laid down. As soon as I laid down, the liquid came gushing out again. My water had broken. Every time I stood up, the baby's head would plug the opening. But when I laid down, it came out again. I called Uche, "You need to leave the pub right now. My water broke."

"Ok, wait right there, I'm coming home!"

I called my parents to let them know that my water had broken and we were heading to the hospital soon. Then I called my friend. "Hey, my water just broke and Uche is at the pub!" I exclaimed, panicking.

"Okay, what do you need? Should I come over?" she offered.

"No, just talk to me right now."

We weren't talking about anything baby-related, we just chatted away until Uche arrived. We had done a birthing class and they had said, "If your water breaks, go to the hospital right away to make sure everything is okay. They may send you home, but just get checked out." I was forty weeks and three days—so three days past the baby's due date.

I was to deliver at a hospital that was a twenty-minute car ride from our house. I went from no pain whatsoever to excruciating contractions in the course of that twenty-minute ride. Gradual labor, be damned.

"Oh my god, this hurts! This *hurts*!" I moaned, with teeth clenched, at Uche as he was trying to drive. We finally got to the hospital and I had another contraction just as I walked in. I keeled over at the triage desk.

"I'm sorry, but we don't have a room for you yet," I was told, while hunched over and trying to make it through a rapidly escalating labor. Finally, they put us in a room in triage and attached me to a monitor.

"Everything's okay," they said. But my contractions were getting stronger and stronger.

It was now 10:30 p.m. and I was five centimeters dilated. I wasn't lying on the bed and I couldn't sit. I stood next to the bed, hunched over, elbows resting on the mattress while I swayed from side to side. Nothing was helping with the pain. Anytime Uche touched me, I was stern: "Don't touch me!" I hated anything he did. He could not come near me. Poor Uche.

The nurse placed a basin in front of me because every single contraction caused me to vomit. I was face down, rocking back and forth and puking. They tried to get an IV in my wrist instead of in the tops of my hands for any medication they might need to give me, but the nurse couldn't get it in. Apparently, I had a rolling vein. By this time, I didn't care about needles, but when she poked me three times and blood started spurting out in sync with my pulse, she finally left to get another nurse.

The next nurse got the IV in within two seconds. Then she came over and started rubbing my lower back in a circular motion with her forearm and some weight behind it for added pressure. I was okay with her doing whatever she needed to do. I liked her. I wanted her to stay with me. But she had to leave and go back to whoever she was working with. As she went, I heard her say, "Oh, I feel so bad for that girl. She's barfing out her baby right now."

Not long after, my room was ready, and I was moved out of triage. I got an epidural right away. I didn't need to be a hero; these contractions were intense. The epidural felt like a little burn to me. They hunched me over a pillow and stuck it between my spine. The anesthesiologist said that because I have a bony spine right where he needed to work, it was pretty easy for him and smooth for me. Then, both Uche and I took a two-hour nap. When we woke up, the nurse team checked my cervix; I had reached ten centimeters and it was time to push.

Uche stood up from the recliner he'd been sleeping in.

"Oh, wow!" one of the nurses exclaimed after seeing Uche's immense height and broad shoulders. "If your baby takes after your stature, I'm not sure how your wife is going to get it out!" Her joke lightened the mood in the room, which had taken on a more serious tone moments before.

The room quickly became chaotic, with nurses and doctors entering from what felt like every direction. Uche stepped out of the way and leaned against the wall behind the bassinet.

"Are you okay?" One of the petite nurses stopped everything and looked at him. "Because if you're going down, I can't catch you. I'll need to get a team in here if you faint."

Uche started laughing. "I'm fine, I'm not going down. I'm just moving back to give you guys room."

I had called my parents to update them when we were ten centimeters dilated, feeling like it shouldn't be long after that until the delivery. But things didn't go as planned. I pushed for a solid two and a half hours, to the point of exhaustion. In the middle of that two and a half hours, the nurse had come in and said, "I'm sorry, but you have to stop your labor. There's another patient who had to have an emergency C-section and the on-call doctor is helping them."

For any woman who's been in labor, they know that to "just stop pushing" is a difficult thing to ask. There is no way. Your body wants this thing out and it is natural to push. Prior to that, they had given me a little pump I could use to up my epidural if I wanted to. I had only given myself enough to take the edge off so I could still feel when I needed to push. When I had to stop my labor, they topped me up completely so I couldn't feel anything.

When it was finally time to push again, Uche and one of the nurses held one of my legs and two nurses held the other. Another nurse was on the monitor to tell me when I was having a contraction and when to push and another nurse put pressure on my stomach to assist in pushing the baby out.

"The baby's shoulder is stuck," I heard one of the nurses say.

I had been pushing so long that the doctor came in and said, "If we don't get this baby out soon, it's going to be an emergency C-section."

They gave me a second epidural, thinking that I was going to have to have a C-section. I was numb up to my chest. At that point, I heard the nurses say, "code." I don't know what type of code it was or what it meant, but I looked up and counted thirteen people in my room. Things escalated quickly; suddenly it was a full house.

During labor, I could only stay on my left side because any time I moved to get into a new position, the baby's heart rate dropped. They had attached a heart rate monitor on its head, which was taped to my inner thigh. Suddenly, the doctor ripped off the heart monitor. I was terrified. She wanted to use the vacuum.

We did not have a birth plan. Our birth plan was to get the baby out in the quickest, safest way for the baby and me. But the one thing we didn't want was for them to use a vacuum. My friends had used the vacuum during their delivery and their son's forehead became purple and filled with fluid. We didn't want that.

"Please, doctor, I really don't want to have to use the vacuum," I said, between deep breaths.

"Okay, we'll alternate between putting the vacuum on just for a bit and letting you push." I'd have to accept that offer, I guessed, because this doctor was going to get this baby out. By then, I had been in labor for a total of fourteen hours. I was pretty done with the pushing thing anyway.

Just before a decision to do a C-section would have had to be made, the doctor—who felt to me like she was elbows deep inside of me, with her one foot up on the bed for stability and strength—gave one last yank and out came our little one! The doctor just plopped our baby on my stomach, with its back to me. *Oh, it's so gunky! But beautiful!* I thought. And perfectly healthy, we were told. *But what is it? A boy or a girl?*

I could have turned the baby over and seen for myself, but I could not bring myself to touch it—it might have been due to sheer exhaustion or the medications causing me to feel foggy, but I couldn't move. It wasn't like in the movies when a baby is delivered and they announce, "It's a boy!" To their credit, now that the baby was safe, the doctors were busy tending to me, making sure I was okay, too.

It got to the point, however, where I looked at the doctor and said, "What is it?"

She said, "Oh, it's a boy," and then kept talking to one of the nurses. Uche and I looked at each other and thought, *Well that was anticlimactic, but yay! We have a boy!* We had wanted a boy—and from the first flutter I could feel, I had had a feeling that's what it would be. We had a name picked out for him. Our little Anson, born at 1 p.m., weighing seven pounds and fourteen ounces, and coming in at twenty-one inches long.

One of the reasons there were so many people in the room is because, as someone who loves teaching dental hygiene students, I agreed to have a couple of medical and EMS students come in, not anticipating any issues. In the end, I regretted that decision—not because of all the eyes in the back of the room staring at my nether regions (again, humility goes out the door in child-bearing), but because I would have preferred to have the doctors be the ones doing all the work.

The difficult delivery meant that I'd need forty stitches to tie me back up. I wish I had drawn a line with watching versus participating; they had one of the students help stitch me up, which at the moment was the last thing I was thinking about. I don't know if it would have made a difference if I had mentioned I'd prefer the doctor to do it—maybe it was because I had just had a baby, or simply because I now had a baby and needed forty stitches—but I am still having issues to this day because of that stitching. Nevertheless...we had our cutie. He was finally here. We were beyond grateful.

We understood why everyone refers to giving birth as "a miracle." It's ridiculous and crazy what women go through in the process. We were in awe and shock and we purposely didn't have anyone come to the hospital so we could soak in the enjoyment ourselves. We wanted this time to be just the three of us. As it turned out, we did run into some friends, though.

After delivery, they wheeled us into the recovery room, where I was, coincidentally, to share a room with Uche's best friend's brother and his wife, who had just given birth! We started sharing delivery stories and realized that the nurse who was able to put the needle in my arm immediately, the one who gave me great back rubs, the one who I didn't want to leave me, was their nurse. Our friend then said, "Oh, you're the one who was barfing out her baby?!" We laughed.

"Yes, that was me." I then realized they were the ones who'd had the emergency C-section; their daughter's cord was in a knot. "Oh, so you're the reason I had to stop my labor for forty-five minutes!" I said.

While we were already really close—their family was like family to us, regardless—now our firstborns also share a birthday, born merely hours apart, right next door to one another.

CHAPTER FIVE:

Recovery and Trying Again

As mentioned, Anson's delivery caused a third-degree tear that required forty stitches. Unfortunately, it got infected, which required antibiotics, and also my bladder prolapsed. I was in such rough shape. To add insult to injury, because of the stitches, I couldn't walk for two weeks or sit normally for eight weeks—I had to sit leaning on my left side. I had a burning sensation down below; if I moved too quickly, the stitching would stretch.

I stayed in bed a lot; Uche would bring food up to the bedroom. I required assistance anytime I had to get up and would have to be held until I could stand on my own. I would venture down to the family room, assisted, for a change of scenery if I could. But getting back upstairs was tough. Uche—or my dad during my parents' visits—would hold me around the waist and help me lift one leg up to the next step, then the other, as I had one arm around their shoulder and the other one holding onto the banister. I was literally taking life one step at a time. It got progressively easier with each passing day.

Once I was able to walk, Uche would still have to help me sit and stand. I couldn't even get in and out of an Epsom salt bath by myself. I had to hold myself up on either side of the bath so I wasn't actually sitting, and then Uche would be there with me to get me in and out. Everything I did required a lot of teamwork and communication.

I may have carried and delivered Anson, but post-delivery Uche had to do pretty much everything for him. When Anson woke up in the middle of the night for a feeding, Uche was the one who got up, changed him, and handed him to me. Anson had his days and nights mixed up, so he would sleep all day and then want to play all night. He also ate a lot. If he wasn't fed every two hours on the dot, it was a problem. Thankfully, Uche was able to take that first month off of work on paternity leave to provide all the support Anson and I required.

Not only did it feel like my whole body was a disaster, but I was also adapting to life as a new mom. I was learning how to breastfeed, which adds a layer of complexity of its own. Anson did really well latching on, but there was a learning curve. Breastfeeding could be painful; my nipples became raw and chapped and they bled for the first few weeks. I had to be in certain positions to breastfeed, either sitting with Anson on a pillow or lying down with him propped into my arm. Holding Anson was the best part of those days; we would just snuggle up against each other, in awe and in love.

As my body gradually sought to gain back function, I spent my days watching movies and daytime television, visiting with my mom, who was retired, and snuggling my newborn. When I was nursing, I would always have snacks within arm's reach. Every night before bed I would stock up my nightstand stash and eat in the middle of the night to keep replenishing myself because Anson was taking all the nutrients.

Because I hadn't been allowed to have sex while pregnant with Anson due to the high risk, Uche and I hadn't been intimate for a year. Once Anson was two or three months old, I tried and couldn't. I had so many complications. Uche never pushed it; he was always supportive. "Let's wait until you're healthy," he would say. I felt horrible for Uche. I wanted that connection with him, but there was no way I could offer it in that form.

I didn't leave the house for the first three months or so, aside from doctor appointments. We didn't have a lot of visitors, but family members and a couple of friends did come by because they knew I was not in good shape. Despite my physical condition and exhaustion (which I think any new parents can claim), our spirits were high. We were ecstatic and euphoric to finally have our baby.

● ● ●

In Jewish culture we do what's called a bris, which is a celebrative baby naming and ceremonial circumcision, that serves as a rite of passage. It is supposed to be done on the baby's eighth day of life, but I wasn't well enough to leave the house to go to synagogue. We asked special permission from the rabbi to wait a bit longer and ended up having the ceremony on day ten—which still wasn't great, but those extra two days helped a lot.

During the ceremony, I sat kind of in the middle, a few rows back with my mom. The event is on the business casual side, and there I was wearing black stretchy pants and a big sweater. When we sat, I had to sit leaning to one side. At one point the rabbi called me up; my mom helped me stand and walk to the front, as Uche was already at the front with Anson. I managed to stand long enough to say our portion of prayers and readings, then hobbled back to my chair with my mom. Uche stayed up front and center with Anson, the rabbi, the mohel (the person we chose to perform the ritual, who was the father of our friend), and my dad.

The rabbi then gave the baby a certificate to confirm his Hebrew name. We named Anson "Zalman," after my uncle—my dad's brother. It's tradition to name a baby after the deceased to honor their soul. I hadn't given my aunt and my baba (grandmother) a heads up before the ceremony; I thought my dad had told the family. When his name was announced, Baba started crying. She was highly honored.

After the ceremony and before the luncheon, I sat for a while in a room with my sister. It's up and down after giving birth. Emotions run high, and I was very hormonal and emotional. I felt I needed Anson, so Jana got him and brought him to me. As that was my first real attempt at walking in public, and it must have been a sight to see, my mom told me later that several of her friends had come up to her, very concerned about me and asking if I'd had a C-section because of my inability to walk and sit very well. At the luncheon, I sat in a chair holding Anson and had people come to me. I didn't work the room. Once it was over, we went home and assumed our position in bed.

I had to learn to let people do things for me after delivery. The good thing about being in a family full of nurses and doctors is we're good at taking care of each other and helping each other out. Jana gave me a lot of pointers on how to bathe the baby and advice on taking Epsom salt baths, nursing and pumping, hormone and feeling checks, and effective swaddle methods. My parents lived within a five-minute drive, so my mom came over quite often to help and snuggle. I just did what I could in each moment. And of course, I wouldn't have been able to get by without the amazing support system of my husband.

Trying Again

Until we started trying again, I felt a peace I had never felt before. We had finally got what we wanted. We were in a new house. We had a crew of friends with babies. We had each other and we had our boy. That peace and contentment lasted until I felt the internal pull for another baby. About a year and a half after Anson was born, we started down the road toward having our second child.

We had three embryos left. We went with the same plan as before. On June 17, 2014, I started taking Estrace again. On June 28, I began taking 200 milligrams of the progesterone suppository. Then on July 3, we did a frozen embryo transfer. We had to thaw all three of the embryos; two survived the thaw, one did not. We had both embryos implanted. We were feeling hopeful again.

One night soon after, we had tickets to see Snoop Dogg and Iggy Azalea at the Cowboys' tent for the Calgary Stampede. I was so pumped! I absolutely love concerts, but Uche isn't an overt concert fan, so when we find one we both would enjoy it is game on. Plus, it was date night! We didn't get many of those.

My parents were watching Anson that evening, so we were over at their house that day when, all of a sudden, I started spotting. It wasn't a lot, but it was there. Right away the mood shifted in the house. I still wanted to go to the concert. I wanted to go out so badly. Iggy was the new "it" thing and gave us the summer anthem that year...I had to see her! I knew no amount of rest was going to prevent what was happening...and maybe it wasn't even happening! Maybe I wasn't miscarrying, and it was just some random spots. I had heard that can happen.

Uche was concerned. I could see my parents' thoughts all over their faces too—in disbelief that I was considering going out, but more concerned than anything. In the end, we made the tough decision for Uche to go to the concert with a friend. Yup, at the last minute I gave up my ticket. I was so mad at my circumstance. I ended up staying at my parents' place with Anson for dinner.

As the night went on, the truth came out. I was bleeding. I was having another miscarriage. Now, we were out of embryos. I was, in a word, devastated.

The more miscarriages I experienced, the quicker I went from, *Oh, dang*, to utter despair. I was frustrated and mad. Each failure to conceive and carry would take a little piece of me every time. It got to the point where, whenever I saw bleeding, I would try to wish it away, as if I could just use my mind power and it would be gone.

Mentally, I kept asking, *Why is this happening to us?* which is a dangerous road to go down. The process was like being on a rollercoaster, with all its ups and downs. During the downs, I would enter an almost hysterical, emotional pit that was very dark. The more those highs and lows happened, the darker that period became. Sometimes I could snap right out of it and rally; other times it took me longer.

When you spend that amount of money and your chances feel taken from you, it is horrible. Losses don't get easier the more you have them. They are all painfully soul-taking. And this one felt the worst because it felt like our last chance. *I'm not going to have any more children. Where do we go from here?* I don't know how to explain the despair I felt, other than I knew I was not complete. I was not done with just one child.

I didn't understand how the embryo transfer hadn't worked, since it had worked for us with Anson not that long ago. *My body knows what to do now,* I had thought. There had been no doubt in my mind. To complete a full round of IVF and have it not work for me more often than it did felt surreal. In my mind, because we were spending so much money and the studies show how effective it can be, I thought it was a sure shot.

We took a little bit of a break to process everything. I contemplated all our options and started the conversation with Uche. The most obvious was trying another round of IVF, which would mean putting down almost another $10,000. An added layer of complexity was that

Jana and Matt had moved back to Calgary, so if we were going to try again with ONE Fertility, it would mean even more money than before because I could no longer stay with them for a month at a time. We ran the numbers and just didn't think we should take that kind of risk.

I felt completely hopeless, lost, and confused. I cried a lot. I had an idea of what my family was going to look like from a very young age and I always knew I'd have multiple children. I had done *everything* anyone and everyone had told me to do. I was healthy, in good shape, ate well, went to all my doctor appointments...there was nothing on my end I wasn't "doing." But my body wasn't cooperating, and no one could tell me why. As my losses continued, the pain and sorrow intensified, but the anger and confusion did too. I was always grateful we had Anson. I still am; he made me a mom, the one thing I wanted most. But I knew he wasn't it for us and I wasn't ready to give up trying. I was convinced we needed to have another child. *We will make this happen*, I thought. *However we can.*

Uche was my rock. He was upset too, but he managed his emotions differently. His usual calm, introverted demeanor was helpful during that time.

It was hard to turn to friends for support at that point because so many of them were having more kids. I enjoyed my friends' kids and celebrated their pregnancies, but it stung more this time. I kept my emotions inside; I would never tell people I was hurting. But now, when people told me they were pregnant, it would take me a couple of days to get over the pain of it not working for me. I was trying to stay positive, but it felt frustrating and gut-wrenching and—to be honest—*unfair*.

I am and always have been, however, conscious of not wanting to diminish the gratitude Uche and I felt for having Anson. From the moment he was born, he brought us such an incredible amount of laughter and joy. We dove into our roles as new parents without hesitation. My mom commented that we were so calm for new parents. We were just so happy he was with us. We would take pictures of him for every little thing; if he had a new expression on his face, picture! If he was sleeping in a new position, picture! If he looked cute snuggling with Uche, picture! We were simply in awe.

We would dance around the house carrying him, prop him on the couch to chill with us, and lay on his playmat together. We would read books and I would sing songs to him; his favorite was "Twinkle, Twinkle, Little Star." Whenever Uche would start singing, Anson would instantly start crying, as if to say, "Daaaaad...just stop!" We thought that was hilarious. When Uche stopped, he stopped crying. When I sang, Anson didn't cry at all.

Anson hated tummy time, so Uche would put him stomach down on his own legs, turn on the TV, and Anson would look up to watch the basketball game...modified tummy time and excellent bonding. On several occasions, we would just watch him sleep, touch his toes, touch his hands, make faces with him...it was magic. We were both extremely hands-on and enjoyed doing whatever it was we needed to do...changing diapers even made us happy.

When it came to having another child, however, we felt completely stuck—until an extremely kind gesture was offered to us that pulled us out of our rut. Uche, Anson, and I were at my parents' house for dinner when they very casually said, "We have something we want to talk to you about."

"Sure, what is it?" I replied just as casually.

"Your father and I wanted to let you know that if you're considering another round of IVF, we want to help you out and contribute to the cost." Clearly, they had been talking about this before because they already had an amount in mind that they wanted to give.

"Are you serious?" I was in shock. Neither Uche nor I was expecting anything like that. I felt a rush of excitement and relief. "You really don't have to do that."

"Yes, but we want to. We are investing in future grandchildren, so it is to our benefit, too," they joked.

Now that I'm a mom, I understand why they offered. As a mom, you want to give everything to your child. You want them to succeed! You want to give them the best opportunities in life. Anything you do has your child's interest at heart. I'm sure seeing us go through what we were must have been hard on them. Maybe they felt helpless, too? There was nothing they could do to control the situation...so this was their way of showing we were supported, we were together, we could do this.

With their help, there was no question we would try again. Much to our surprise, we decided we would go back to the clinic in Calgary, even though we didn't love it. It was in a new location and had been updated since the last time we were there. Greens and taupes colored the waiting room area, professional pictures of families and their babies were hanging on the walls, new comfy waiting room chairs were put in place, offices were down a hall with floor-to-ceiling glass doors. It was more open and welcoming than before. I was adamant about getting a different doctor and we did, and he was more caring. I liked him a lot better. I felt like maybe this could work. When I told him where we were at and what was going on, he empathized more. I still didn't love how the clinic ran and how it wasn't very personal, but it was a better experience than our first one there so we moved forward with it anyway.

We decided on a full new round of IVF. I don't think we realized how tough the IVF process was until I went through it a second time. The first time, we were going through it blindly. The second time through, I remembered, *Ah, yeah this is a lot*. But we wanted another baby for us and a sibling for Anson more than anything.

We started the whole process again. On January 10, 2015, I started with two injections of Gonal-F and Luveris. Then January 14, I took 0.25 milligrams of Cetrotide®, which is the medication that prevents premature ovulation. (I was on Suprefact at the other clinic, but this medication does the same thing.)

On January 19, they put me on 10,000 IU of the hormone HCG. This was similar to the Ovidrel, which helped make me ovulate. On January 21, we did the egg retrieval. The egg retrieval process in Calgary through the Regional Fertility Program felt much more clinical. To begin with, the waiting area was a big room with several private areas around the perimeter. Each area had a recliner chair, another chair for a significant other, a locker for our belongings, and a drape we could pull across. It seemed like there were ten couples occupying the seating areas. It was packed. In the center, there was a common nurse station and doctor station. We would stay in our area behind the curtain until we were called to the procedure room. I was wearing a hospital gown and little socks. Uche waited for me back in that little area with the curtain pulled.

The procedure room was big, open, and white. I was on a cold, metal hospital operating table with a thin cushion and a hospital blanket. At ONE Fertility, the room had been plusher and had a bed with nice sheets. Here, it wasn't very intimate like the other clinic had been. The lights were dim, but they weren't warm; turning lights off in a stark room doesn't make it any more inviting. Also, during my retrieval at Regional, the staff and doctors were all men—not that this is a bad thing, but when dealing with such an intimate women's issue, it is nice to have feminine energy around, whether that is through having female staff or a room with a feminine touch. I missed the emotional connection I'd had with my female doctors and nurses; they had told me every step of the way what they were doing as they did it. ONE Fertility was cozy and comfortable, like a hug. Everything was done slowly, with intent and with comfort and warmth; it felt like family, rather than a doctor-patient relationship.

At Regional, the male staff used a very logical and methodical approach that didn't feel inclusive. They just went through each step as though checking off a list. The doctor's movements were quick and strong. I had a little discomfort but was told we were almost done. The whole retrieval seemed super quick. I was a bit more sore after this round, too—it could have been because of the doctor's different approach or because my body had done this before and wasn't a fan.

After the retrieval at Regional, they wheeled me back to be with Uche because I was under conscious sedation. We waited until I was able to be more mobile and then we went home. Once again, nine eggs had been retrieved. Seven were fertilized, the same as the first round. Still, we realized our chances were not as high, so we decided on intracytoplasmic sperm injection (ICSI) again for an additional $1,500.

However, after five days, only three embryos survived, versus the last time when all seven did. We were told the news over the phone. I felt concerned because our chances were lower given the number of embryos that survived, but the egg quality was higher this time, so it almost canceled the worry out. I had three great-quality embryos!

On January 26, we did a fresh cycle transfer. We only put one embryo in because the quality of these embryos was so high. It paid off. I got pregnant. And I knew from the start that it was a little girl.

CHAPTER SIX:

Heartbreak in Hawaii

WE WERE IN MAUI FOR MY FRIEND CARLY'S WEDDING. I WAS eighteen weeks pregnant. It was May 6, 2015, and we were at the bride's bachelorette party, which was a snorkeling cruise. I had permission from our doctor to travel, and permission to go to the bachelorette party, but because I was on modified rest, I wasn't allowed to swim. I had a floating belt and a boogie board ready, so I could bob in the water while the others went snorkeling.

The boat was open with benches all around the sides and a few rows of benches in the middle. There were around fifteen of us on the tour. Most of us had known each other for years or had at least heard about each other on many occasions so it was like we knew each other. We sat around laughing and joking with each other, enjoying the beautiful day.

"I can't believe you won't give me any dirt on Carly," the wedding's MC teased me. "You've known her the longest, you must have some good stories."

"Sorry, I can't think of anything incriminating. (I absolutely could.) But if it'll help you, I'll write a little something up and speak at the rehearsal dinner tomorrow night."

"Really? That would be great. I was hoping a few more people would come forward to speak."

I didn't move around on the boat much; I stayed in my seat, talking to those around me. Once we got to our snorkeling destination, we were given a briefing and instructions about the location, where to snorkel, and the equipment. One by one, everyone got their gear on and hopped off the back of the boat into the water.

I put on my belt, my mask and flippers, and took a boogie board. I didn't rush. I was one of the last ones off the boat. Very slowly, I lowered myself into the water from the ladder at the back of the boat. No jumping in, no big movements...I just glided. Everyone went their own ways, swimming around and laughing.

I hung around close to the boat, bobbing in the water.

"Oh, wow, a squid!" I exclaimed, surprised by my quick find. "That is so cool!" I looked up to tell my friend, but it was gone before she could see it. A few moments later, I felt a pop in my lower abdomen, similar to twisting a muscle in the neck. My excitement at seeing the squid turned to panic. *Oh no! What was that?*

I carefully floated over to the boat and slowly got back on. I put my equipment away, sat down, and waited for everyone else to come back. A few people were on the boat, including Carly's mom, so we chatted a bit, but

I mostly sat quietly resting. *I wish everyone would get back*, I thought. I was ready to go ASAP.

The ride back seemed faster than the ride out. Everyone was having a good time and the vibe was chill. My panic started dissipating as time went on. I wasn't in any discomfort and I had no other symptoms.

I was anxious, still questioning if I should have been out there at all, but I talked myself through the fear, saying I would be fine because I was barely moving. The ocean and water have always been a source of tranquility for me, and I tried to focus on letting go.

The next day, Uche and I were at the pool when I felt pressure almost like a period cramp, but lower, throughout the day. There was no bleeding, no cramping, no fever, no indication that anything was the matter. I convinced myself it was the muscles stretching with the baby growing.

That evening, we were in our small but modern and comfortable condo, getting ready for the rehearsal dinner. I was about to get dressed when what felt like a balloon started to come out of me. I panicked, went to the bathroom, and called for Uche to take a look. There was no blood, but there was some sort of sac starting to fall out of me.

"I think it's the baby," he said, very calmly. I could tell by the look on his face that this was serious.

"What?" I went into complete shock. The tears started immediately. I was upset, confused, not sure if he was right...he had no idea what he was looking at, but what else could it be? I wasn't in physical pain, but absolute despair. *No! Not again!* I didn't want to believe it. My whole body crumbled and my soul was crushed.

I went and laid on the king-size bed and didn't move. Every scenario was playing in my head...the pop, the pressure that day. I was going over *everything*, analyzing it all. I was mad at myself that I didn't go get checked after the pop feeling; I was mad at myself for not getting checked out for the pressure feeling; I was mad I went snorkel bobbing; I was mad at everything I had done.

Uche quickly got the phone and called me an ambulance. He was downstairs with Anson while he called, and I was upstairs bawling in bed. I called Carly to let her know what was going on and that we wouldn't be at her rehearsal dinner. She quickly ran over to her mom's condo and put her mom—a retired doctor—on the phone. When I explained what was happening she very calmly said, "This doesn't sound good. What condo are you in? I will come over and help."

"There is absolutely no way you are missing your daughter's rehearsal dinner for me. I will keep you updated. Besides, we are pretty far down the road from you, at a different property." I was incredibly touched by her concern. The ambulance showed up fairly soon after I hung up.

The EMS couldn't bring the gurney into our room because the hallways were too narrow. They called the fire department and five firemen carried me out lying in a yellow blanket, to the ambulance.

Uche and Anson were not allowed in the ambulance because Anson needed a car seat, so they couldn't legally transport him. We also didn't have access to a car at that time. Uche tried to find someone to watch Anson but ended up having to arrange to get a car and bring Anson along with him to the hospital—a forty-five-minute drive away—to see me.

When I arrived at the hospital, thoughts started flooding through my head. I continued replaying my day, questioning why I didn't get checked out if I'd had pressure, why I went on the boat. I analyzed every little detail, wishing I had done *something* differently.

Once Uche and Anson got there, I put on a brave face for Anson, even though I had tears in my eyes. It was a complete sham. I was lying through my teeth, telling him I was okay when I was not okay, but I didn't want him to pick up on anything being wrong.

They did an ultrasound and my uterus looked like an hourglass. I'd had several ultrasounds in the past and knew it looked wrong. They rushed me up to obstetrics (OB), where the doctor said that my cervix had completely dilated. He consulted with other doctors and specialists to try and find options, but really, there was nothing they could do. They had to induce labor, and I had to deliver the baby. Uche had been right; the "balloon-like" sac he had seen was the baby's amniotic sac.

"Please, don't. I will lie in this bed forever. Just don't take it out." But they couldn't do that. They sent me to labor and delivery right away.

We ran into another problem then; children weren't allowed in the labor and delivery room. The entire wedding party and all the guests were at the rehearsal dinner, on a cruise ship, and not set to dock until later that night. Uche left to take Anson back to the condo, where he'd have to stay until the guests returned.

They broke my water and gave me meds to induce my labor. Then, I just had to wait. I had never felt so alone. No one was in the room, aside from a nurse who would occasionally pop in and check my progress. I had no way to contact anyone since amidst the chaos I'd left my phone back at the condo. I had a TV in my room with "Saturday Night Live" on. The show was playing every single Justin Timberlake episode on a loop. I just sat there watching them. I was too distraught to move or change the channel. I was numb.

During one of the nurse's quick visits, I told her I had to go to the bathroom. "Is it okay if I get up?"

"Yes absolutely," she said. I had a private room with a small bathroom, so I just got up in my gown. The walk over seemed as normal as it could be. Nothing alerted me to what was about to happen. What came next was probably the hardest moment I've ever experienced in my life, and the one I remember most vividly.

I used the toilet and when I went to wipe, I felt my baby's tiny little feet hanging out of me. I wasn't in labor; there were no contractions. The baby was mostly in, but partly out. I could not believe what I was seeing. I was beside myself. I remained seated, holding onto the railing on the wall for further support, bawling my eyes out. I reached down and wiped off the feet; I wanted to touch them. When I was able to get up, I washed my hands and took a quick look at my red, puffy, crying face. I couldn't look at myself for long. Before I left the bathroom, I lifted my gown and took one more look at my baby. My heart was broken. And I still had to deliver.

I laid back down on the bed. Then labor hit. The nurse came back in. I started having contractions and just as I had with Anson's delivery, I got really sick. I vomited with every contraction. At 10:07 p.m., I finally delivered the baby—a little girl Uche and I had decided we would name Ashtyn.

I started bawling more as the nurse swaddled her up and put her in a little bassinet on the other side of the room. Uche made it back to the hospital at 10:35 p.m.; he walked in, went over to the bassinet, fell to his knees when he saw her, and began crying heavily. I've never seen him like that before or after; it was so hard to see. Everything happened so fast, we weren't able to offer each other much by way of comfort, either.

"Do you want to hold her?" the nurse asked Uche, quietly and compassionately.

"No. I can't," he replied. He took a step back. He was quietly processing what had just happened and could barely get any words out.

"Rena, would you like to hold her?"

I wasn't sure I wanted to, but I made myself because I knew down the road that I might regret it.

"Yes, please," I replied. The nurse placed her softly in my arms. She was so tiny. Tears streamed down my face and landed on our little girl's forehead. I went to wipe them away, but because she was so little, her skin wasn't totally formed yet, so it was sticky. She looked identical to Anson; they were spitting images of each other, with the same nose, forehead, and lips. I couldn't believe it. *She was developed enough to look like our son.*

"Do you have arrangements for her? Do you want to take her with you?" our nurse asked. I could barely comprehend her questions. I wasn't thinking straight, I was so emotional.

"What do you mean, take her?" I asked.

"Some religions and some people will take the baby to bury it or to hold a ceremony."

I was so mad at the time that I was in this situation, that I answered for Uche and me without even thinking, "No, you keep her." She ended up at the morgue at Maui Memorial Hospital, and I think about that decision every day.

After that, I got rushed in for a dilation and curettage procedure (D&C) because we were traveling in two days and the doctor wanted to be certain that my placenta wasn't retained. The surgical procedure is performed after miscarriages to remove the uterine lining. This would make sure I had birthed everything and avoid any further complications.

As soon as I got in the operating room (OR), my body started convulsing uncontrollably; I think it had to do with the rush of emotions and the trauma. It was a lot. I was shaking. I couldn't control it. The OR nurse put a heating cover over me, held my hand, and I went to sleep. When I woke up, I was groggy and Uche was gone.

I asked a nurse where he was and all she said was, "Oh, he left." Then she left the recovery room. I was still waking up from anesthesia, with *Why would he leave me?* running through my mind. Then I started getting upset that he'd left, especially in a situation like this, and I couldn't understand what had happened. I also had zero concept of what time it was. I found out later that he had been kicked out at midnight because visiting hours were over. The nurse didn't explain any of that to me.

I barely slept that night. Uche and Anson showed up first thing in the morning, around 6:30 a.m. I was surprised and elated to see them walk in. When I was by myself, I was hysterical and bawling, and as soon as Anson showed up, it was like a switch turned on. I put on a brave face. It was so Jekyll and Hyde, so fake, but I didn't want my little man to see me like that. Plus, it gave me a break from my misery and offered me some brightness in my day.

The doctor who delivered Ashtyn came to check on me. He was acutely empathetic. "My wife and I lost a baby at eight months along," he shared. "Things will get better with time." At that moment, I didn't feel it at all. I didn't feel like anything was ever going to get better. My whole world had just crashed. And I was still second-guessing every single move I had made up to that moment.

We left the hospital in a wheelchair with a bag that had Ashtyn's birth announcement, her footprints, a pink blanket, a knitted baby cap, and her ID bracelet, but no baby. We were completely broken and empty.

Uche carried Anson as I was wheeled out to the car. Naturally, Anson had a lot of questions. He was concerned about me and wondered if I was okay. We kept our answers very simple, without any details. Uche did most of the answering because I was in an out-of-body state. We told him that the baby stopped growing and wasn't in my tummy anymore. We told him he had a sister. He was so proud. We told him her name. We showed him her blanket and tiny footprints. He was just over two years old at the time, so the severity of what was going on obviously didn't register.

When we got back to our room, the wedding was about to start. I started thinking that we should go to the ceremony. We had come all this way. I laid down on the bed and picked up my phone; I still had a little time to decide. My friend Kylie had texted me earlier in the day, not knowing what had just gone down. I decided to call her back for emotional support. Even before she answered my FaceTime call, I had already started bawling again. When the video came on, she saw my wretched face.

"Rena, what happened?!"

I just cried and shook my head no. That's all I could do. She understood immediately. She started crying, too. Uche went over and played with Anson to give me some privacy. I told Kylie every detail. She was in shock, and I think I still was, too. She knew my struggles and everything we had endured up until then. She had been so hopeful for us, and I could tell this news shattered her. When we hung up, I started organizing my things to go to the wedding.

"What are you doing?" Uche looked up at me and asked.

"Getting ready for the wedding," I replied.

Uche was firm, "We can't go."

I said, "Yes, we can. Let's just go, and we'll stand at the back so they can't even see us." Anson was scheduled to be the ring bearer with two other boys. "We'll let Anson walk down the aisle."

I was pretty adamant that we should go. We had flown all the way to Hawaii, Anson was having his debut as a ring bearer, we had paid for the trip, and I didn't want it all to be a waste. I was experiencing high and lows, elated one minute and a puddle of tears the next. Hormones do crazy things to you. Uche put his foot down. "We're not going to go." In hindsight, I'm glad he said we shouldn't go. I would have been a hot mess.

Two days after the wedding, we flew back home to Calgary. I moved in with my parents to spend some time healing and to avoid facing memories in the house where we had thought we would soon bring home our new baby girl.

CHAPTER SEVEN:

Grief and Support

AFTER WE GOT BACK FROM HAWAII, I WAS DIAGNOSED WITH cervical incompetence, which happens when the cervix completely dilates without signs or symptoms. The only way to know you have it is to experience a preterm birth. When we lost Ashtyn, it was the absolute worst and darkest time of my life. The other miscarriages I'd had paled in comparison, by far.

What felt like a saving grace at the time was a complete change in environment. Uche had recently been promoted at work and given the opportunity to transfer to Houston, Texas. We had been looking for an opportunity to leave Calgary. I never thought I would live in Texas, but the opportunity came up and we welcomed it. We were ready for a new adventure, something different.

I had no part in packing up the house; Uche handled everything. I was too enmeshed in my grief. We arrived in Texas and moved into corporate housing. I didn't know anyone, and no one knew me or what we had just been through. And I didn't have the constant triggers; we weren't in our house, so I didn't have Ashtyn's room to look at all the time. We weren't around our friends, who had thought I was pregnant and super happy. I could remove myself from the situation. However, I realized later that I did not grieve properly because of the move. I distracted myself with logistics—not just of the move, but of our next steps as a family.

One of the most amazing things about the Jewish culture is that no matter where you go, you can always find community. It's one of my favorite parts about the faith. So, when we moved to Houston, one of the first things I did was find the Jewish Community Center—it's an instant family. I had reached out to the director before we moved; every Friday is our Sabbath, and the center holds a *"Tot Shabbat"* program, which is specifically designed for families with children ages birth to kindergarten. Parents bring their toddlers, sing songs and do prayers, light candles and eat challah, and just schmooze. I felt the need to go for myself, and also for Anson, who needed to meet kids his age. However, Uche surprised me by coming with us that first Friday. He is not Jewish, so I leave it up to him to decide what he wants to participate in. I was comforted knowing he wanted to come with us. It was a change, and we all enjoyed it.

The corporate housing we were living in during our first three months in Texas happened to be by a mall, so I would take Anson to the mall every day to play on the play structure. I was very good at putting on a brave face around him. No one would have known that I had so recently lost a baby. Anson never saw my grief. I was always there for him. I took him swimming, to the zoo, to play groups. I never missed bath time or bedtime. But once he was in bed, the darkness encompassed me.

As soon as Uche came home from work, I would pass Anson over to him. Once Anson was in bed, Uche and I would sit together, have a few drinks, and eat fried chicken sandwiches—which is not usually my jam, but I did whatever I needed to do. Some nights that would be enough, and I could just go to sleep. But other nights Uche or I would grab another bottle of wine and I would lock myself in our beautiful, big, walk-in closet and sob uncontrollably. I did this every single night for about a month.

What made the situation even worse was that my body didn't know the difference between delivering a full-term or preterm baby. Just before we'd moved to Texas, when I was staying at my parents' house, I was in the shower when I felt an odd sensation in my breasts. I called for my mom and she came in the bathroom to explain that my milk was coming in. It felt different this time. I had all the symptoms post-birth that a term pregnancy would have. I was speechless and taken by complete surprise. Just when I thought I was at a manageable place in healing my trauma, reminders like this would happen. *I should have a baby with me now!*

I went through a range of emotions during this time: mad, sad, angry. I experienced a lot of triggers and often I couldn't predict what the triggers were going to be. I would see a pregnant woman and hate her, which is not at all my character. Or I'd see a bird doing something super random, and it made me think of a bird I saw in Hawaii and then, all of a sudden, I was right back there, reliving the trauma. Smells would even trigger a memory. There was no rhyme or reason to when it would hit, but when it hit, it was like a freight train I felt I could not get off.

Fortunately, I wasn't working at the time. When we moved to Texas, I was not licensed to work there yet, and I was in no mental or emotional state to get my license. I stayed home and focused on Anson.

As a way to keep me going, I started researching surrogacy—only sixteen days after losing Ashtyn. I was still determined to have another child, and I was feeling pretty desperate. I started Googling "surrogacy" in the United States and around Texas. I called a few clinics and they broke down what was involved and the pricing. I learned the difference between surrogacy in Canada versus the States. In the U.S., surrogacy is big business. I was quoted $95,000-$100,000. There was another catch—we wouldn't be able to bring our embryos across the border.

After I got the U.S. price, I called the Calgary clinic and got an overview of the process and the costs involved there. In Canada, it's not legal to compensate or offer compensation to a surrogate (although there are some reimbursable expenses). That's why finding a surrogate is so hard in Canada. We had friends in Canada who had been searching for a surrogate for five years. If we did find a surrogate, the costs were essentially the same we had incurred before—the thawing of the embryos, implantation, medication, etc., plus the cost of hiring a lawyer.

I wrote out a brainstorm/flow chart of our options and what could happen next. Later that night, Uche and I were in the bedroom when I shared the chart with him.

He knew from the start he didn't want to go the adoption route. Then he looked at the price of surrogacy and politely shut that option down. At the thought of trying to get pregnant again, he hesitated.

I come from a medical professional family. My family members are doctors, nurses, dentists, dental assistants, and hygienists, whereas Uche's family are mainly engineers and Information Technology (IT). In order to survive, I needed to keep going and determine my next step. Uche, on the other hand, was more analytical.

"Sit down," he said. I sat next to him on our bed. "Can you just see what your body has gone through these past few years and take a minute?" He looked directly at me. "I don't think you should try and get pregnant again. Look what you've gone through. Look what we've gone through. I don't know how healthy this is for your body." He had never said anything like that before. That changed the tone of our conversation. To that point, I had never considered my body. I had not put it into that perspective. He continued, "I'm done. I am emotionally tapped out and I've put enough money toward this."

Up until this point, he had gone along with everything I had researched and proposed we do. He had never been really firm about anything. We had always been on the same page. This time, when I was going through our options with him, he was present, but I could tell he wasn't into it like I was. His shoulders slumped and he said, "I have my son, I don't need to go another route and I don't want to."

And I wouldn't listen. I was adamant. "No, this has to happen. We're having another baby." We left the conversation with me saying, "Well, we still have two embryos, so I'll just do it. I'll get implanted again."

The way we handled things was very different. Uche admits he does not understand what I was going through. It's natural to have different perspectives because first, it was my body, and second, I had been pumped with so many hormones, then had a baby, then went through everything that happens to your body after having a baby—the stitches, milk production, the sheer exhaustion—it's a wild ride. The pull to be snuggling a newborn was still so strong.

Husband's Perspective: Uche

When we began this journey, I wanted to let it happen naturally. My mindset was, *Let's let everything progress how it does.* But it's not Rena's personality to let things happen by chance. She needs to be in control of what's happening.

In Hawaii, when she wanted to go to the wedding, I said, "You cannot go to the wedding in that state. There's no way. We are going to stay together as a family and we're going to mourn." In my mind, that was the right thing to do. I realized that something traumatic had happened that we needed to deal with. Since she's so strong-willed, if I don't say what I'm thinking and convey that to her in a way that makes sense, she's going to go forward and do what she wants to do.

We would have these discussions where we'd talk about our infertility journey, and she would say, "I understand what you're saying, but we need to be pregnant by December." Then she'd plow forward, whether I liked it or not. That's just her personality, and it's fantastic, I love her for it. But after Ashtyn, she was fatigued. She was running on fumes and I could see it. At some point, I had to say, "I'm done with this," to let her know that the mission was indeed over and that she needed to pick up another cause to fight for. And in my mind, that cause was Anson. He's beautiful.

I was worried that Rena was missing out on some of Anson's childhood because her focus was so directed toward having another child. I tried to tell her, "If we only ever have Anson, we can still have a beautiful life. The three of us together are amazing. We would be able to travel and do all types of things that we wouldn't if we had a larger family." I tried to show her some of the positives of having one child.

Emotionally, the loss and the entire process wore at me. But I was able to compartmentalize, which is my personality. I would say to myself, "We've gone through this event," and then close the event and move on to the next phase of our lives. Rena, on the other hand, would relive every moment. She would pinpoint a specific moment and focus on it, replaying it over and over again in her mind. It haunted her. I wouldn't go through those types of scenarios in my mind, so I didn't get it. I didn't feel all of those emotions because I wasn't going through the same thought process.

Furthermore, it wasn't my body going to the doctor visits, so we men tend to be a little bit detached from the experience. But at the same time, I never said to Rena that she "should get over it" or "just forget about it and move on." I let her go through the emotions that she was going through, even though I didn't understand the level of pain that she felt. To this day, on Ashtyn's birthday or due date, Rena will get very emotional, whereas I'm sometimes oblivious. Her grieving process is ongoing; it's so ingrained in her whole being compared to me.

As for me, I feel I had adequate support. If I had felt along the same lines as Rena, maybe I would have been a bit deficient; it would have been hard for both of us to support each other, especially after moving to Houston, where we didn't have any family to support us.

I also had work as an escape; I was busy starting a new position in a new location. That distraction kept me busy and helped me through it all, in a way. Rena provided support for me too because when I did have to come in and support her, we would go through the emotions together at that moment. That process allowed me to release whatever pent-up emotions I had when trying to help her.

●　●　●

My close friend from high school, Carla, and I had drifted apart and hadn't talked in fifteen years. She had seen on Facebook that we'd moved to Texas and private-messaged me. She and her husband were transferred to the same city two weeks after us! So, we all met for dinner one night. Carla is a very excited, expressive, lively person, and I firmly believe she came back into my life when I needed someone like her most.

We met at Cyclone Anaya, a Tex-Mex restaurant. Tex-Mex is big in Texas. We picked that spot because it was one of the few places we knew at the time, as Uche and I had been there before during one of our scouting trips. The restaurant has a nice green space with turf where kids can run around and play, so we figured it was a nice place for both our families.

We found our parking spot and were making our way to the entrance when I saw Carla and her family walking across the street. She had a big smile and was waving her hand crazily at me. I was waving back.

"Hello-o-o-o!" she called out. We darted across the road and threw our arms around each other. We stood there hugging for what felt like forever, leaving our husbands to have to introduce themselves to each other. When we finally let go of each other, we made our way to the restaurant door. We had been deep in conversation, catching up, when Carla glanced at my belly.

"And, we have a baby coming soon!" Carla said. I had told Carla prior to our move that I was pregnant. This was an innocent statement, but nothing could have prepared me for those innocent declarations, and my insides seized up and dropped.

All I could muster was, "No, I already had her." The look on Carla's face said it all. No one knows what to do or say in situations like that, so I tried to play it off. "Don't worry. There's no way you would've known, but we can get into that later," I said, and we kept moving along as I held in my tears. We sat at a high-top table, with all the adults on one side and Carla's two children and Anson on the other. The kids got along immediately.

Carla ordered a mule, and the rest of us ordered the big Beergarita—the house-size margarita that requires two hands to drink, with a beer dumped inside it. Conversation was easy for everyone, as if we had all known each other for years. I have no idea what we talked about. I just know it was a smooth conversation and we all got along. After dinner, we went out to the green space. While Uche and Carla were playing soccer with the kids, I sat with Carla's husband Shaun, whom I had just met, having a drink and chatting. It was the most fun I had had in a very long time.

Our families started hanging out regularly after that, and I opened up more to Carla. At one point she said to me, "I have no idea what to say, and I might never know what to say, but I'm always here and I'm always listening." We all need a friend like that, but especially under circumstances like these.

She may have felt she didn't know what to say, but she knew instinctively what to do when I'd have my break-downs. For example, we were at the zoo one day, when all of a sudden, I started crying uncontrollably. I'm not a hysterical person; I can keep myself in a box if I have to, but sometimes, I couldn't keep control and the tears were automatic. She mobilized into action, taking the kids to look at an exciting animal in the opposite direction from me, so I could have my moment.

Her support didn't stop there. She helped me unpack in July when we moved out of corporate housing and into our home. She helped me with Anson. She let me cry. She let me be mad. She played with the kids regularly. She took the kids around our new city. She became family.

One thing I learned is that when we need support, we find our people. We might not be actively searching; they may find us. And they may not be who we expect them to be or who we think they should be. And that's okay. We need to bless and release that, too. Holding onto the desire for certain people to be there for us when they won't or can't just becomes toxic.

I've also learned that it's unhealthy to ask ourselves, *Why is this happening to me*? It is such a hard question, one that many people going through this experience face. At the time, I often felt like life was very unfair. People would make off-hand or insensitive comments that they thought might help. I once had a dental patient comment to me, "Well, you're not getting pregnant because you're not sixteen or in a bar or on a one-night stand." Well, why can this sixteen-year-old get pregnant and I can't? I was on a lunch break one day and there was someone living on the streets who looked like she was eight months pregnant and wigging out on drugs. I walked by her with my eyes welling up thinking, *I could offer a child something so great. I don't understand why the world is doing this to me.*

It's natural for these questions to go through our minds, and we will constantly doubt our bodies and wonder why. It was hard for me to tell if the feeling was valid or just grief, but I thought my body was failing me—that it was my fault. Uche would tell me, "You can't think like that. This isn't anything you're doing wrong." He said that I just needed to focus on our goal, that thinking about the whys and the ifs and what-ifs leads to a rabbit hole down a darker path. He was right, of course, but I couldn't hear it at the time. I am a very strong-willed person; I want what I want when I want it and it doesn't matter what anyone says to me. Looking back, all of what he said was thoughtful and true.

Now that I have gone through this experience myself, I would say it's important to feel every emotion that comes because they are true. It is human nature to feel guilt and resentment in situations like this; my suggestion is to not suppress or repress those feelings, because that only makes it worse. Feel those emotions, but only indulge in them for a brief period of time. Then, focus on where you are headed. In other words, let negative emotions come, but then let them go.

Uche was more positive than I was, initially. I feel and think of everything negative right away. When I started going into the dark and getting upset, asking "why me," he was great at reminding me that other people's story wasn't our story. "And who cares if so-and-so is pregnant?" he would say. "It doesn't affect us. Let's look at what we're doing." He focused me in on us and the positive things happening with us. We did have our amazing son, after all. Having someone (who may or may not be one's partner) who can support our feelings as well as redirect them in a positive direction if we are unable to do that for ourselves is really helpful.

Our support person with whom we can feel safe and share authentically doesn't have to be our partner, a family member, or even a friend, however. We can always find our people. It could be a hairdresser, or a grief support group, or someone we hire, such as a therapist. It could be a friend from high school who you haven't talked to in fifteen years.

Friend's Perspective: Carla Rutz

Rena always says I saved her life, but she doesn't know how much she saved me right back. My husband and I had just relocated from Connecticut to Houston, Texas with two children under five and I didn't know a soul there. When I found out Rena and Uche were also moving to Houston, I felt ecstatic relief. *Yay, I will have a friend!* Anybody will tell you, a cross-country move like that takes some adjustment. Moving to a new place is so scary because you have to start all over again rebuilding your network, your support system, your entire life. I was grateful for Rena. We spent every day together; our kids played together and we were each other's lifeline. Rena and I built our lives together in those first months together in Texas—it was her and me, supermoms united!

When supporting a friend or loved one experiencing infertility or related struggles such as a preterm birth, here is what I have learned: Many people are so afraid of saying the wrong thing that they don't say anything at all, which is worse. If you don't know what to do or say, here are ways you can support them:

1. **Read**. If a situation is uncomfortable or you don't know enough about it, read about it, learn about it, then talk about it. The more I read and hear stories from people who have been through a particular situation, the more that helps me offer the right kind of support for my friend.

2. **Don't forget the men**. Men need support, too. First, make sure the man is equipped to support his partner. Once you know the woman has a support system in place, look at who is supporting the man and how you can support them.

3. **Never ask about pregnancy**. In conversations, let them bring it up if they want to talk about it. In general, don't ask questions that are none of your business. Their emotions and capacity to deal with the situation vary, and you have no idea whether this is something they are willing to talk about at that moment.

4. **Pick your moments.** At the same time, you don't want to avoid the topic or conversation altogether. Read a room and know whether

this is a conversation for right now. A crowded restaurant or a large group is not that moment. Be careful not to bring the subject up immediately, and to wait for the appropriate moment and then make sure they know you're there for them.

5. **Any emotion and every emotion is okay**. Reassure them that what they are feeling is normal. It's such a personal journey and everyone's experience is different. Feelings and reactions are complex. Grief is grief. You have to let it be.

6. **Let them know you are there for them**. Most mothers who have experienced a miscarriage or preterm birth want to know that you're not moving on without this child; you are moving forward with them in love. Let them know: *We're not going to forget your baby.*

All of these situations will vary depending on the depth of your relationship with this person. I hope this gives enough perspective for you to support a friend through any stage in her fertility journey. Rena and I had each other to get through that initial shock of living someplace new. Texas was so different from any other place either of us had ever lived and we figured it out together. We both benefited from the bond of close friendship, advice, and being each other's day-to-day touchpoint.

CHAPTER EIGHT:

Surrogacy

I HAD A DOCTOR LINED UP TO TAKE OVER MY OB CARE ONCE we moved to Texas. I called to let her know I had already delivered, and she wanted to see me anyway. She was very sweet. I didn't know her at all, but as soon as she walked into the room during our first visit, she hugged me. She wanted to do a hysteroscopy, which is an in-office procedure under conscious sedation. The procedure allows the doctor to look inside and inspect the uterine cavity using a hysteroscope, which is a narrow telescope with a light and camera at the end. It is inserted through the cervix and inside the uterus. I had the exam on August 17, 2015. That is when she discovered my cervix wasn't closed in its natural state. She didn't have to dilate it to put the scope in. I also had a fibroid, as well as a prolapsed uterus.

A fibroid is a noncancerous growth in the uterus that can develop during a woman's child-bearing years. Some symptoms include heavy menstrual bleeding, prolonged periods, and pelvic pain—and in some cases, there are no symptoms. I didn't have any symptoms, but to create the best possible environment for getting pregnant, the fibroid would have to be removed. Depending on their size, fibroids can go away on their own, but other times they need to be surgically removed.

A prolapsed uterus means that my uterus wasn't in the position it should be in; it had fallen and was hanging low. "You are still able to carry a baby, but eventually you will need a hysterectomy," she said. "Also, due to your age, I would get it done here before you go back to Canada." In Canada, performing hysterectomies for women of child-bearing age is not typically practiced. In an emergency, that's another story, but mine did not fall under that category. That latter part, I filed away for later—it was the first part of what she said that I couldn't get out of my head.

She said I could carry another baby.

I got back in touch with our doctors and turned frantic again. I called the clinic in Calgary, where our embryos were still being stored. I got all the information I needed about how to move forward, when I would have to travel, what medications I needed, etc. I was ready and Uche was not.

I still had this deep hole inside of me—a feeling that our family wasn't complete. Uche didn't understand that and was more than happy with just the three of us. I was incomplete.

● ● ●

It was a sunny day in August 2015 when my phone rang. I didn't recognize the number, but I decided to answer it.

"Hello?"

"Hi, Rena, this is Melissa."

"Oh, Melissa, hi! What a nice surprise!"

I had met Melissa through my sister. They worked together at Canadian Blood Services in Ontario. While I was living with Jana and Matt during my treatments, we saw a lot of Melissa. She and I became friends too. Melissa had been with Uche and me on our journey to get pregnant from the first day we started at the Ontario clinic and knew about all our past experiences.

"I hope I haven't caught you at a bad time, but I just heard the news about your little girl through your sister and I wanted to reach out." She had sent a message to Jana wondering about a dress my sister had lent her for her daughter; she wanted to give it back in case I was having a girl. My sister let her know that I had already delivered Ashtyn.

"My heart breaks for you, Rena. I'm so sorry. I want to help in any way I can, and that's why I'm calling. I want you to know that if you and Uche want to try surrogacy, it would be an honor to be a surrogate for you."

My jaw dropped to the floor and my eyes teared up. *Did she just say what I think she said?* She seized on the silence to continue.

"Shaun and I are done having our own children, so this is something I want to do for you."

"I...I don't know what to say..." my voice trailed off.

"You don't have to say anything right now, just think about it, talk it over with Uche, and let me know."

I couldn't wait to tell Uche. I was on cloud nine, completely in awe of the generosity my friend had just conveyed. Uche immediately agreed—it's not every day someone offers to surrogate for you.

"But," he said, "this is going to be our absolute last chance at having a second child. If this doesn't work out, there is no more trying, okay?" He was done financially and emotionally, but he was willing to give surrogacy a try. How could we not? A surrogate just fell in our laps out of nowhere!

I called the Calgary clinic to tell them we had a surrogate. I was shocked when they said they wouldn't allow us into the surrogacy program. We still had two frozen embryos; I didn't understand why we couldn't do it. "We want you to try again yourself," they said. It felt like they were pushing me to try to get pregnant, and I didn't want to. I told them that having a preterm baby had been hard enough and I didn't want to go through that again. By now, I'd had seven miscarriages through the different stages: one during the naturopath stage (which I didn't know was a miscarriage until later); during my first embryo transfer of IVF, I miscarried those two embryos. During the second embryo transfer, I miscarried one and kept my son. During the third embryo transfer, I miscarried those two, and then I had Ashtyn. Even though I delivered her, she is considered a miscarriage because she was only eighteen weeks. While I was lying in the back of an ambulance in Hawaii, the friendly EMS man had told me that twenty weeks is the cut-off for survivability and for doctors and nurses to be able to help a baby along.

They did not listen—not even the managers or the head of the surrogacy program. They would not let us in. I had never considered that we could be denied this chance. It felt like we would get two steps forward and then a brick wall would get put in front of us. This is the first time I agreed with what Uche had said about my body not being able to handle another preterm birth—I couldn't handle it emotionally, either. Now we had a surrogate, but no clinic.

I decided to call ONE Fertility and see if their answer might be different. We had to wait several weeks for an answer; management had a meeting, then they checked with the licensing board to see if it was okay, then they were worried about us not residing in Canada at the time. We ultimately got our lawyer involved to help answer questions for them. I was so desperate at this stage, and time was my *worst* enemy when going through fertility treatment; I was impatient and wanted everything done ASAP.

But to our great relief, when they got back to us, they said yes—they'd do it! The clinic in Burlington actually worked out better because Melissa lived close by; we wouldn't have to worry about flying her to Calgary. *Everything happens for a reason*, I thought. We weren't meant to be with the Calgary clinic at all. I was so happy; we were one step closer to having another child.

Having Melissa surrogate for us at ONE Fertility wasn't a walk in the park. We had to arrange for a transport company to move our embryos from Calgary to Burlington, for another thousand dollars. It was very stressful because if anything happened to those embryos in transport, we were done. That was it. There was a lot riding on this transfer and my anxiety was in full gear. Thankfully they made it to Burlington intact.

Our fertility lawyer wrote up a detailed contract between us and Melissa, outlining some things we never would have thought about. It stated that once Melissa had the baby, it belonged to Rena and Uche; she was not going to assume parentage of this baby. It answered questions such as, does Melissa hold the baby first, or does Rena get to hold the baby first? If Melissa has to take off work, what portion are we going to cover and what portion is unemployment insurance going to cover? It even outlined restrictions for Melissa—she was not to have any part of her body pierced or tattooed or to touch a cat litter box during pregnancy. We flew to Toronto to meet with Melissa and sign the contract.

We tried to make an intense experience a little fun. When going through in vitro and embryo transfers, sex schedules are dictated by the doctor. As a surrogate, this process affected Melissa's relationship with her husband, Shaun, because they weren't allowed to sleep together. We were informed by our lawyer that in general, surrogates aren't allowed to sleep with their partners in the event that they get pregnant with their own biological child. Makes for a messy situation. So, we bought him a blow-up doll as a joke, to keep things light. They laughed; they were very supportive of the whole process.

We kept our surrogacy plan a secret from everybody, except for the people involved. We did not tell our families. We did not tell our friends. We did not want to hear anyone's opinions, and we didn't want to burden anyone. I say "we," but it was really me—I didn't want anyone to know, and Uche respected that.

A Message from Above

One of my consolations during the very difficult period after losing Ashtyn was an extremely vivid dream I had about a month after moving to Texas. I woke up crying, thinking it was real. My Uncle Don, who had passed away from ALS several years prior, came to me in my dream. We were walking along Palliser Drive in Calgary, which is close to where I grew up. He had his arm around me and all of a sudden, he turned to me, hugged me, and whispered in my ear, "Don't worry, I've got her. You're going to be okay. Everything is going to be okay." I shot up in bed.

Anytime I had a bad moment, I would think of what my uncle said to me—Ashtyn was with him. I don't consider myself an overly spiritual person; I do have faith, but this was on a level that I had never experienced before. The dream was so real that it moved me into a deeper belief system. I started to believe that things happen for a reason, and I started to believe in miracles. I have not had a dream like that before or since. But I do believe that there's something higher up there, and that is a comforting thought.

I had another spiritual experience several months later, after we had moved from Houston to Austin. When I say we tried everything and left no stone unturned in our fertility journey, I mean it. What started as a joke ended up having a significant impact on my grieving process. I would never have thought I would be someone who would go to a psychic medium, let alone write about one, but here we are.

When we first moved to Austin, I met a mom and her two boys in the park, and our boys connected. It turned out she worked for a medium, who also happened to be her best friend. I told Uche about her and he bought me a session with the medium as a playful birthday gift.

He thought the gift would be lighthearted and fun, but it turned into so much more and gave me the closure I needed to get me out of my rut after having Ashtyn. I was instantly able to cope.

The session was over Skype. A couple of spirits came through first, one of which was my zeida (grandfather) who I have never met. That was cool. She then told me to think of the name or the relationship I have to the person I want to connect with. *My daughter.* Ashtyn's spirit came flying in. The medium knew everything, including things that only Uche and I knew. For instance, we always have a pot of purple flowers on our front porch. Purple is a color that both Uche and I associate with Ashtyn; we came to it separately and happened to talk about it one day. When we see something purple, we think of her. The medium said Ashtyn knew about the flowers in front and said, "Thank you."

She also commented that Ashtyn was laughing and saying, "Daddy doesn't get it. He's trying really hard, but he doesn't understand what you're going through." She also commented on the bedroom upstairs in our current house. Nobody knew, at the time, that it was a storage room. She said that Ashtyn went in there and blessed the room and knew it was for her sister. I was taken aback. For me, the fact that she knew the room was upstairs, and the fact that she said "sister" brought me a great deal of comfort. We had just gone to Toronto to sign surrogate papers a couple of weeks before; this was a dream.

The medium told me that Ashtyn's spirit kept buzzing around her head. "She's like a little spitfire," she said. Everything she described about her made me think, *she sounds a lot like me.* Then, as though reading my thoughts, she said, "She's a lot like you."

She went on to say that Ashtyn had a heart condition. The spirits had gotten together and decided it would be much easier for us to handle her passing in this manner versus her being alive for six months and then passing away. "Heart condition" didn't mean anything to us until a year and a half later, when Uche's brother passed away suddenly from a genetic heart condition. We knew nothing about it at the time.

The medium also predicted there was going to be another baby. She said, "You absolutely are going to have another child, but it's not from you. I see legal documents handed to me, which means adoption, or something." I told her we had just signed documents for a surrogate. This reassured me we were on the right path.

Then they started talking about Melissa, our surrogate. The medium said that Ashtyn really liked her and thought she was so nice, but started giggling and said, "But she's going to cheat. She's not going to be allowed to eat certain things, but she's going to eat them anyway." (I later told Melissa about that; she chuckled and said, "Yeah, I totally would.")

The medium also brought up my uncle, Don, about whom I'd had the very vivid dream. She said, "The picture I have of him in my mind is of him sitting on the couch, hanging out, watching TV. And Ashtyn is all over him, buzzing around." The fact that she knew about the flowers, knew about the room, knew about a heart condition, knew about another child, and knew about Uche not understanding, literally was everything we knew.

When I talked to Uche about it, after the fact, he started laughing and said, "It's true. I really don't get it." And that was the first time that Uche and I sat down and had a conversation about how his process of dealing with the loss was different from mine.

Surrogacy Procedures

On June 15, 2016, Melissa was set up to do her first frozen embryo transfer. The cycle was canceled by the doctor because, due to the fertility medication she was on, her uterus was not an optimal environment for the frozen transfer to happen. On July 4, she was set to go for another cycle, which was canceled again for the same reason. At this point, they started adjusting her medications to see why she was reacting the way she was. Melissa was one of those women that could look at her husband and get pregnant. But when she was put on the fertility meds, it caused issues. She had fluid in her uterus. Her lining wasn't thick enough. We had to keep postponing implants. To me, another brick wall.

The next scheduled transfer date, September 11, was also canceled because of a lab issue. The way the embryos were frozen in Calgary was different than the way they froze them at the Ontario clinic. They needed to bring in an outside lab technician who knew how to thaw the embryos the same way they were thawed in Calgary.

Finally, we were able to do a frozen transfer on October 26. They put one embryo in, and it didn't take. At this point, Melissa said she needed a break because Christmas and New Year's Day were busy times for her and her family, and she wanted to make sure she was in a good place for the pregnancy to happen for us. So, we agreed to wait until after the new year.

Once we were on our very last embryo, Uche sat me down and said again, "I can't do this anymore. I am emotionally and financially tapped out. We have a son, and he's great. If this doesn't work, we're done." That's when I knew how serious he was about this being our last shot. I understood that pushing so hard for the second child was my doing because I knew I needed it. I told myself, "I have a fantastic son, who we are learning is extremely athletic for his age. Maybe our time, energy, and money are supposed to be focused on him and his athletics." For the first time in nine years, I let it go. I surrendered control completely because there was nothing else I could do—our first embryo didn't work with Melissa, we only had one left, and Uche was done. On January 23, 2017, Melissa had the right uterine conditions, and a frozen embryo transfer was completed. That was our very last embryo.

CHAPTER NINE:

Miracle Baby

TWO DAYS AFTER OUR LAST FROZEN EMBRYO WAS TRANS-ferred into our surrogate, Anson, who was only four at the time, was scheduled to visit the doctor for an x-ray of his spine. Since I was planning to go in with him, I had four different nurses at four different times ask me if I was pregnant leading up to the appointment, to make sure it was safe. Of course, I said no.

"Are you sure?" they pressed.

"Yes, I'm sure."

"Okay, but you're going to have to sign a form when you get here in order to accompany him into the room."

"No problem."

The day before the x-ray, I counted how long it had been since my last cycle just to make sure, since so many people had been asking me if I was pregnant. *Hmm, that's strange*, I thought. *Forty days*. That was the longest I had ever been without my period, so I decided to take a pregnancy test just to rule it out.

I was on the phone with Carla at the time. I thought nothing of taking the test while on the call. All of a sudden, I saw the word PREGNANT. I don't know what noises I made, but Carla said, "Oh no, what? What's going on? Is everything okay?"

"I'm pregnant," I said in disbelief.

"Wait, what? Melissa's pregnant?"

"No, *I* am," I replied.

It was very confusing. Even Carla was confused. "Uh, one second," I told her. I reached underneath the bathroom sink and pulled out a stack of tests. I took another test: positive. Took another test and another test. Four tests, all positive.

"Holy crap, Carla, I'm really pregnant!"

She was screaming and I was screaming and I kept repeating, "This isn't real." I didn't believe it; never even once in a million years did I think I could get pregnant naturally.

"I need to tell Uche!" I said. "He's not going to believe it."

"Okay, go, go! I'll call you later," she replied. But I didn't want to be alone.

"No, no, no, stay on the phone with me. I need you on the phone while I drive." Uche worked twenty minutes away, and I knew I needed to tell him in person. Carla stayed on the phone with me the whole time, but I was in shock. I didn't even know what to feel because it hadn't sunk in yet.

I had never shown up at Uche's office unannounced. I called him from the car. "Uche, I'm outside your office. Can you come down here for a sec?"

"I can't come down for a coffee right now. I'm about to go into a meeting."

"That's fine. I just need two minutes of your time. I'm in the parking lot."

He came down and sat in the front seat of our car. He was confused. All I did was hand him a positive pregnancy test while crying. He looked at it and said, "Whose is this?" I looked at him again, and he said, "This is yours?" And I said, "Apparently."

We were speechless and in shock. He canceled his meeting and we went for lunch.

Looking back, I definitely had symptoms, but I never associated them with pregnancy, and I could justify every single one. I had big boobs, but I thought my cycle was late and I was brewing a big one. A late period was not unusual for me. Our shower smelled like mildew and it was really bothering me, but no one else could smell it. We even had two people look at it to rule out mold. Also, I was falling asleep midday. Anson would be playing, and I'd pass out sleeping, and I'm not a napper. I didn't associate any of that with pregnancy.

I made an appointment with our doctor, and she confirmed the pregnancy, though we didn't yet know how many weeks along I was. She said my levels were so high, that it was possible I was pregnant with twins! I started freaking out because if I was having twins and Melissa was to get pregnant from the implant, that was a whole lot of babies happening! I called Melissa immediately after that doctor's appointment and told her the news.

We laughed; all of us were in shock. Of all the scenarios we had discussed, this NEVER crossed anyone's minds. There were two weeks to go before we could find out if Melissa was pregnant or not. In those two weeks, I started realizing I didn't know how I was going to manage it all. Melissa was in Canada and we were in the United States, possibly having two babies at the same time. I didn't know how the logistics were going to work. We decided we had to tell our families.

I FaceTimed my mom, and then my dad. Normally I would have called them together, but my dad happened to be out of town on a guys' trip. We hadn't told our families about the surrogate yet, so I started by telling her about Melissa and she was excited.

"Oh, that's great," she said.

I continued. "Yeah, it is. Melissa got implanted and we're really excited, but just so you know, you're going to be a nana again anyway, because I'm pregnant." She went silent and didn't say anything for a long time until I said, "Aren't you going to say something?" She was in such shock. It was a lot of information for her to process. I was expecting an over-the-top crazy reaction, so when she simply froze, I said, "Okay, well I'm going to let you go. We'll talk again in a bit."

After we hung up, I looked at Uche and said, "Well, that didn't go how I wanted it to." I called my dad next, and when he answered the phone, I asked him if he was in a room by himself; I didn't want anyone else around. He was, so I told him about the surrogate and then I said the same thing, "You're going to be a papa anyway because I'm pregnant." I saw his jaw drop; he took the phone and turned it around in a circle, so we were all spinning. He made it really fun. He was so surprised and excited; it was a great moment together. Next, we called Uche's parents, and they were ecstatic.

After my dad got home from his trip, I called my parents again, and this time it felt like a big celebration. After some time to process the information, my mom was thrilled, understood what was going on, and said not to worry, that if Melissa ended up pregnant as well, they would fly over and be with Melissa and the baby in Canada while we were handling the baby in the U.S.

As it turned out, that wasn't necessary. Melissa did not end up getting pregnant. Nevertheless, I tell her all the time that the only reason I got pregnant was because of her. When we passed our last embryo on to her, I truly let go of control. And that's all I needed to do.

Surrogate's Perspective: Melissa Button

I have a daughter and twin boys and was on maternity leave when I reached out to Rena. When I heard she had lost Ashtyn, I was heartbroken. We FaceTimed and Rena updated me on their situation. There I was, sitting with my two babies and my daughter, loving up on them. I wanted that same experience for Rena. I talked it over with my husband and told him I wanted to offer to be their surrogate. Even before I finished, he knew what I was going to say. He said, "Go for it. Let's see what's involved."

I will say that becoming a surrogate required a lot more preparation than I thought it would. A lot of it had to do with Rena's embryos being across the country in Calgary. I had to have more testing than I had expected, have an IUD (intrauterine device) removed, then a hysteroscopy, and then have the IUD re-inserted, and then months of planning and testing. Logistically, there was a lot of back and forth. The fertility center in Burlington was a thirty-minute drive from where I worked at the time, and I was working different shifts. The back and forth of getting bloodwork and going for the procedures and follow-up appointments was a lot to manage. Months of hormones made me feel crazy. It took some time for my cycle to regulate.

My husband was super supportive throughout the entire process. He was not so keen on the times when we couldn't have sex but that is understandable. It was a long time, especially when we kept having to postpone the procedures, and then we would have to start over again. It was taking more time than we had thought and it was stressful, especially with the added hormones.

Being a surrogate was like a roller coaster. I felt a range of emotions: excitement, nervousness, stress, worry, joy, and relief. I wanted it to work so badly for them that it caused me a lot of additional stress. I went through two rounds of embryo transfers, and the first one didn't take. When I didn't get pregnant, I felt like I'd let Rena and Uche down. When we found out Rena was pregnant after the second round of embryo transfers, I was so surprised and excited for them. I was also nervous. Rena and I being pregnant at the same time added a different layer of complexity that we couldn't have predicted.

The idea of me having to possibly look after and bond with the baby added a level of worry that being their gestational carrier didn't: *What if I have one of their babies in my tummy? How will I bond with that child if I do end up having to look after it? What am I going to do if Uche has to be with Rena... raise the baby for a little while?* All of those things started swirling through my mind. It was a strange situation to find ourselves in.

I found out shortly after the procedure that the second round didn't take. Part of me continued to worry about Rena's second pregnancy. I kept in touch throughout her pregnancy in case they needed me. I like to see things through to completion. It felt weird in the end to have gone through all of that preparation and planning only to have it not work out the way we had planned. Of course, it worked out as it was meant to, but it felt odd and incomplete for me to not actually have been their surrogate. Rena and I spent so much time focused on making it work that it was a let-down to not be able to see it through. There was a period of adjustment for me; I wasn't sad, but it felt like this period of my life was all of a sudden over.

In hindsight, there are only two things I would have done differently:

I wouldn't have put the IUD back in. Taking it out and putting it back in caused two strong surges of hormones which caused and continue to cause ongoing issues.

I would have worried less. Surrogacy is expensive, so a big concern was that it wouldn't work. I wanted to help them fulfill this dream of having a second baby.

If you are considering surrogacy, here is what I would say to you:

1. **Find someone you trust**. It is a very intimate and high-stakes process.

2. **Consider a surrogate with similar values.** Be clear from the beginning whether the surrogate is going to be involved in the baby's life. If the two families plan to stay close and involved in each other's lives, it may be important to know you parent the same way and share similar parenting philosophies. What happens if you choose to raise this baby in a way she wouldn't? Is she going to be okay with that? That came up in our situation and I never would have thought it would.

3. **Clear communication is key.** All parties involved, spouses, and significant others must be included.

4. **Establish legal contracts.** Legal boundaries are crucial. Everyone is clear on their roles, and there are contingencies in place. If something were to happen to you, to the surrogate, to the child, or to the parents, what measures are in place?

5. **Make sure all parties are on board.** If the surrogate has a spouse or significant other, make sure they support this choice and process.

6. Be in it for the right reasons. I remember people asking me whether I would have a hard time letting go because I had carried the baby, but I didn't have that sense. To me, it was Rena and Uche's baby all along. It would have been different to give that baby up at the end, but it was never a concern of mine. I was never in it for money or for any other reason than to help Rena and Uche.

At one point during the contract process, my attorney said, "This is where you ask for the things you want. If you want yoga classes or for them to cover other expenses, ask for them now." I was shocked. I wasn't going to take advantage of them. That's not what this was about. I just thought I had a good house to make a baby.

7. Understand the process, before you decide. Understand everything that needs to happen. We had to go through psychological assessments. We were all so worried, as couples, about those assessments. In hindsight, it is kind of funny. We were all stressed about the assessment when really, it was a friendly little man making sure we were in it for the right reasons.

Rena and I were in touch constantly during the process, but with us all having busy lives and raising children and working and living in different countries, and now with a pandemic, it's easy to drift apart.

● ● ●

I did my research and booked myself with the best high-risk OB doctor in Austin. I had a copy of my chart from the Calgary fertility clinic, and I also had kept my chart from the emergency room in Maui. I brought all of that information to the doctor's office and told them all about my history. His nurse seemed like she was writing forever. Then he came in and put his hand on my shoulder and told me, "In my twenty-five years of practice, you take the cake." We had a laugh over it, and I said, "Please tell me this isn't twins. I can't handle that surprise too."

He did an ultrasound. I've had so many ultrasounds that I could see for myself that there was only one sac. I said, "Phew, there's only one." He laughed and said, "You can probably read these better than me now." The reason my levels were so high was because I was already nine weeks along!

We set a date to tell people, aside from our parents, that I was pregnant, but the date came and went. I kept pushing it back. I was not ready. We were still in disbelief; I wasn't ready to go on that emotional roller coaster or expose myself to the vulnerability and potential of having to explain myself if the pregnancy didn't go to term. I didn't even want to buy anything for the baby until I was pretty far along; sometimes I stopped myself from feeling excited, as a subconscious way to prepare myself for another failure. It was very hard to enjoy the journey when every little thing caused me to worry.

Unless someone was with me and saw that I was pregnant, they wouldn't have known. I was all belly, so I would strategically place my son in front of my stomach or place myself so my lower half couldn't be seen when posting pictures on social media.

The way we told Anson that I was pregnant was by bringing him to the twelve-week ultrasound. He sat in a chair against the wall next to Uche while I laid on the bed.

"What are we doing here?" he asked, confused.

"It's a surprise," I told him. The ultrasound technician came in and started the exam. Uche and I knew what we were looking at right away. I felt a calm of relief when I saw her.

"Look at the TV, Anson. What do you see?" we asked.

"I don't know," he replied.

"Look, that's a baby in Mommy's tummy. You're going to be a big brother." He was surprised and excited, and shocked, and all the good things. We all had huge smiles on our faces. Then Anson got quiet all of a sudden. I could tell he was processing.

He asked, "You have a baby in your tummy? But how did it get there?" I looked at Uche and he looked at me. We froze! We weren't prepared for that question yet.

"Uh..." is all we could say. Then the ultrasound technician jumped in and said, "It's magic!" Anson was amazed.

"Wow!" he lit up. Thank goodness for that technican. She saved us.

"It's a girl, right?" Even though I knew the answer to this, I asked it anyway. Just to make sure. This is the first pregnancy we found out gender pre-delivery. Getting pregnant was surpise enough.

"It's a girl!" I knew it!

I was really sick from weeks nine to fourteen; I was barfing everywhere. I was on bed rest for the entire pregnancy. I significantly limited activity, rarely went out, and didn't lift anything. I would take Anson to and from school, but Uche would take him out to the park and to baseball practices. I was on high alert all the time; any little tweak or twinge made my thoughts race.

The doctor told me I needed to have a cerclage, where they stitch the cervix shut, so I wouldn't have another preterm birth. This surgical procedure usually occurs at thirteen weeks. At around eleven weeks, I felt a drop and a pressure down low, and I started having flashbacks of how I felt with Ashtyn. I ended up in the emergency room because I was not going to ignore the feeling this time.

Thankfully, the baby was okay; the OB on call said the drop I felt was my prolapsed uterus. They placed a cerclage in a week early at twelve weeks, on March 13, 2017. I was in the operating room, where they gave me a spinal injection, which is like an epidural. It's conscious sedation; I was lying on a table with my legs in stirrups, and they used a speculum and put in a stitch. It took only twenty minutes. The baby was a scheduled C-section with no option for vaginal delivery based on my previous complications. Plus, with my prolapses, we were worried that pushing would affect things more.

I set milestones for myself. *I just need to make it to twenty weeks, then I can relax a bit and tell people I'm pregnant*, I thought. But then when I got to that milestone, I'd make a new one. I welcomed any symptom because it told me I was still pregnant. I couldn't be anywhere near the kitchen when food was being prepared, or I would get sick. Uche was in charge of making dinner while I hid out in our room. I craved milk, bacon and candy.

When I had been pregnant with Anson, I felt the hard part was over and I could sit back and enjoy my pregnancy bliss. This time, I wouldn't allow myself to fully appreciate the pregnancy because I was expecting something to go wrong. I tried my best to enjoy it, but I was constantly aware of the "what ifs." Once I was finally in the third trimester, I felt the realness of it and some of my fears subsided, although I knew I wouldn't be at total peace until I had her in my arms.

About a month before the due date, I'd asked my doctor if he would tie my tubes during the C-section, which was very weird, given how long we had been trying to have kids.

"Are you sure you are not having any more babies?" he asked.

"Yes, I'm sure." I was finally done going through what we had been through. I didn't want to be a forty-year-old who ends up with a surprise baby; I could only handle one fertility surprise per lifetime, and Uche felt the same.

"Okay, as long as you are sure." I am sure.

The cerclage was removed at thirty-seven weeks, and as soon as they took it out, I was automatically three centimeters dilated, so my doctor understood why Ashtyn essentially fell out. Despite my dilation, I ended up carrying our second child to thirty-nine weeks. The day before the scheduled C-section, I checked into the hospital. Mom had come into town early and stayed with us for almost six weeks, in case I went into labor early, so she helped watch Anson.

After my labs, they took me to the operating room. The anesthesiologist stands out in my memory; he was so compassionate and sweet and talked to me the whole time and even held my hands when Uche wasn't there yet. I was given my epidural and prepped for surgery. I was completely numb up to my chest again. This time, they laid me on the operating table and everyone moved me because I couldn't move myself. A big blue sheet was placed across my chest so I couldn't see what was happening. That's when Uche arrived, geared up in a one-piece gown and a scrub cap.

Uche sat in a chair next to my head on my left. I could also see the doctor, the anesthesiologist, the nurses, and the doctor's assistant—five of them in total, as opposed to the thirteen I'd had with Anson. The doctor was talking about his kids coming home from college, which was a weird experience because here I was in surgery, but the doctors and nurses were talking about their kids and carrying on conversations about everyday life.

Our doctor asked if Uche wanted to watch, which he did. He talked us through the procedure as they went along. There was a lot of pushing and pulling on my body.

"Okay, now you are going to feel a lot of pressure, as if an elephant is on top of you," the doctor warned. He did the best he could to let me know what was coming, but he was rightfully more concerned with the surgery itself, communicating with his crew, my health, the baby's health, and a successful delivery. He would peek over and ask me, "How are you doing, Mom?"

It was very sweet and loving in an operating room setting, which is very dichotomous. It was a clinical setting, with its bright lights and cold table, but the whole experience was so much more enjoyable than when I delivered Anson because I wasn't having painful barfing contractions. Plus, Uche was with me and we got to talk through the whole thing.

"Can you see what's going on?" I asked Uche, who was taking pictures. He could—and when I later saw the pictures, I was glad I could not! The sheet is there for a reason and I'm happy it was there; essentially my insides were all out.

Before our baby was delivered, the doctors asked what her name was because they wanted to put it on her bassinet. "Can I tell you when she's born?" I asked. In my head, it was important to wait until she arrived. I have no idea why, but it was a strong feeling. After everything we had been through, I just didn't want to jinx or mess anything up.

"Yeah, no problem," we were told.

Our daughter's birth was less climactic than Anson's because she was simply lifted from my belly. Like before, there was no big announcement of, "You have a baby girl!" or anything of that sort; they were too busy tending to both the baby and me. But when I heard her cry, that was enough for me—I started crying, too. *Wow, she's here. And she's healthy!* It was the best feeling in the world. At that moment, I had the feeling of being complete. This was my family. I felt it instantly.

Arisa was born at 7:46 a.m. She was seven pounds, five ounces, and twenty inches long. Our pregnancy announcement ended up being Arisa's birth announcement. When I made our new addition official on

Facebook, many people commented that they never knew I was pregnant; we had told so few people.

Arisa was even more "gooped up" than Anson. The "goop" is called Vernix caseosa; it's a white, creamy, naturally-occurring biofilm that protects the newborn's skin. Uche held her first, then she was placed near my head and shoulder for a quick snuggle before the nurses took her away. I don't know if this is a difference between C-section and vaginal births or the difference between American versus Canadian processes, but as soon as she was born, they took her to the pediatrician and checked her out. Uche went with her, so I was left alone with the doctors for about an hour while they were stitching me up.

Again, the anesthesiologist was incredible. I was excited and full of emotion when Arisa was born, and then when Uche left the room with the nurse and Arisa, I was really confused. I felt lonely.

"Where's my baby? Where's my husband?" I asked. It felt like it was taking too long; I didn't understand what was going on.

"Your blood pressure has gone up a little bit," the anesthesiologist said.

"Well, I'm kind of nervous. Where did my baby go?"

"Don't worry, she's being taken care of. Do you want me to hold your hand?"

"Yes, please, would you?" He sat there and rubbed my hand and talked to me. Since the birth, no one had asked our baby's name, so when I was talking to the anesthesiologist, I asked, "Do you want to know her name?"

"Yes, I really do. What's her name?"

"It's Arisa." I felt better just saying her name.

"Wow, that is the most beautiful name ever." That gave me the connection I had been hoping for with the anesthesiologist because he was the only person on my side of the curtain. I am so grateful to him for supporting me in that way.

Once I was stitched up, I was wheeled into the recovery room, which was just an area with a curtain. I was there for what felt like forever. Then, suddenly, the curtain opened and there was Uche with the nurse, pushing Arisa in her bassinette. I felt a big emotional rush of, "Oh, there are my people! I'm so happy to see you guys!" Uche gave Arisa to me right away. I held her on my chest and didn't let her go. Here she was, and she was mine. Arisa latched right away.

Anson was in preschool at the time and my mom had picked him up early that day. After Arisa was born, we called her and she brought Anson to see us. I was in bed holding Arisa when he came through the door.

"Hi bud," I called him over. "We have a surprise for you."

"What is it, Mom?" He was so confused because he'd never seen me in a hospital bed before. He walked around the bed, took a look at Arisa, and said, "My baby."

"Yeah, your baby's here," I said to him. He was so excited.

My mom had teary eyes and helped him into bed with me. "You can't touch Mommy's tummy but come see your sister."

We had to stay in the hospital overnight to be monitored. In Canada, I'd had to share a room after delivering Anson, and Uche was not allowed to stay. But in the U.S., I got a private room where I was able to rest right away, and Uche could stay and spend the night with me—which turned out to be beneficial because complications arose later.

All of my friends in Canada who had had C-sections were only given Motrin and Tylenol to manage any pain. For me, the nurses pushed taking narcotics. It didn't feel like I was given an option. This may, again, be a difference between the U.S. and Canada. They put me on Norco, which altered my perception; the walls were covered in purple, patterned wallpaper. My mom was in the room as well, and at one point while I was nursing Arisa I turned to my mom and said, "I'm really high right now."

"What do you mean?" she asked, confused.

"Those purple spots are moving. Can someone please hold Arisa for me?" I was scared that Arisa would get high from my milk.

A nurse was called in, and we explained the situation to her. "Don't worry, only a very small amount of the drug passes to the baby and it won't affect her," she said.

"No, if I'm feeling like this, then it will impact her, too," I contradicted the nurse. I knew what was right for my baby.

In the hospital room, there was a whiteboard where the nurses would mark my pain level every time they came in. I was never above a five; I usually hovered around a four or a three. I realized that was because I was on so many meds, which I am very sensitive to.

"I don't want narcotics," I told the nurse. "I only want a Motrin."

"But we need to be ahead of the pain," I was told.

"I'm not in pain, I'm feeling high. I don't want this."

"Okay, we will half your dose," she reassured me.

Later during the night, when it was time for me to get up and start walking around, I made it to the bathroom and looked in the mirror. I was so pale that the color of my lips matched the color of my skin. "Oh, crap, this isn't good," I said to myself. I turned to go back to the bed, thinking *I don't feel well.* The next thing I knew, I was waking up to Uche screaming my name in my face and three other nurses surrounding me. I had passed out.

When we had a nurse shift change, we found out that the nurses hadn't halved my dose. They were still giving me full doses of the narcotics. At that point, I was done with the hospital. My doctor came in and I told him, "You need to discharge me. I don't want to be here. I want to be at home. I'm being given medications that I don't want."

I didn't realize until then how much we have to advocate for ourselves in the U.S. system, versus the system I was used to in Canada. Knowing what I know now, I wouldn't have even taken one pill.

After having Arisa, I ended up with a prolapsed uterus, bladder, cervix, and rectum. My pelvic floor muscles were so weak that my bladder was pushing my pelvic floor down. Everything to do with that region was uncomfortable. I couldn't engage with my kids as much, like jump on the trampoline or run. Any time when I contracted the muscles in my abdomen, my insides jarred. It was a really weird feeling. Sex was very uncomfortable. If I had to go to the bathroom, I had to go immediately—holding it was not an option.

To try to manage the situation, I was placed on pelvic floor therapy for nine weeks. This entailed having a tiny vaginal probe inserted, which emits a very low-grade electrical signal to excite a set of nerves and muscles in the area. The muscles contract with this electrical signal, which in turn makes them stronger. Or that's the intent anyway. It reminded me of a Transcutaneous electrical nerve stimulation (TENS) machine, which is a method of pain relief involving the use of a mild electrical current. I would lie there with this machine inside me for half an hour.

I also had to do kegel exercises daily on the hour, where I'd hold my pelvic muscles for ten seconds and release. I couldn't always do it. However, none of these exercises helped, so my doctor said the next step was a hysterectomy. On June 12, 2018, I had a laparoscopically-assisted vaginal hysterectomy.

Although I had already gotten my tubes tied, a hysterectomy felt more definite and permanent; my uterus was being removed. It was a certainty that I had no possible way of having children ever again. Even though I didn't want any more children, I felt like a part of my femininity was being taken from me. On the flip side, I was so excited to never have a cycle again, and that outweighed everything else. The way I chose to look at it was to kindly tell myself, "You've been on this intense, crazy up-and-down journey. This is the final stop and then it's done."

For the procedure, I had two small incisions on either hip and another one in my belly button. A camera was inserted and the surgeon watched the image on a TV in order to perform the procedure. He took out my cervix and my uterus but left my ovaries because of my age;

they didn't want to put me into early menopause. I don't get a cycle, but I still have hormones. He also pulled up my rectum along with my bladder to keep them where they need to be. When they were done, they pulled out so much gauze from my abdomen that my body felt like a clown car. It just kept coming and coming. I was also pretty bloated because they had put air into me as they were doing the procedure.

A hysterectomy is typically a day surgery. We went in the morning for what was supposed to be about a two-hour surgery and a two-hour recovery period before going home. It's never that simple. I had a reaction from the general anesthesia. I was pretty sick, so I had to stay longer. After a hysterectomy, you have to be able to use the washroom and expel a certain amount before you can be discharged. I tried once and failed. On my second try, I did it! We were free to leave. It was 4 a.m. and I had been there almost 24 hours.

The average recovery is four to six weeks, but I was grateful to be feeling pretty good after two. I had an eight-month-old, so maybe I forced myself to feel better. I still had to watch the incision sites and be careful walking. I couldn't walk upstairs, and I couldn't drive for a while. There are a number of rules to follow to hasten the recovery, but my mom was there for a long weekend to help me out, so recovery wasn't so bad.

Finally, we had put an end to our fertility struggles. Our nine-year journey was complete. We had our family. I felt a massive weight lifted off me. We didn't have to think about clinics anymore. We didn't have to think about money anymore. Any bonus my husband got didn't have to go to fertility—he decided what to do with it. Up to that point, I'd had it planned out before he even got it. We would schedule treatments around his bonuses. To have that off of our plates felt like a big escape; we could finally just be.

CHAPTER TEN:

The Fruits of Our Labor

EVERYBODY HANDLES MOTHERHOOD DIFFERENTLY. THERE ARE working moms, stay-at-home moms, part-time working moms. I was a working mom up until we moved to Texas. And since we've been here for the past five years, I've been a stay-at-home mom. I am the type of person who, when I do something, I give 100%. I gave 100% when trying to get pregnant and now I give 100% while I'm raising my kids. Every ounce of my being is going into them right now.

When I was working full time, all I wanted was to be a stay-at-home mom. And now that I'm a stay-at-home mom, I want to work. When both of my children are in school, working part-time will be the perfect balance for me. I used to always think the grass is greener on the other side. Now the thought will still cross my mind, but then I catch myself and reaffirm, "No, my situation is what

I make of it." We've been fortunate that I haven't had to go back to work; it has been by choice that I'm home with the kids and it feels like the best choice for our family right now. After the kids get older and I go back to work, I'm sure some of my identity will come back because I will have something that is just for me.

There's a perception that motherhood is a magical role. And it is, but that perception is not entirely painted in reality. The truth is, it's very hard. It's difficult to prioritize self. It's draining. A friend of mine described motherhood as hard and heartwarming, exhausting and exciting, we are lucky and they are loved. I agree with her sentiment completely. Uche is great at prioritizing himself. But as a women, we naturally care on a level that is different from men. I have a constant list running in my head making sure everyone is taken care of before I get to myself. For a time, it felt like there was no Rena anymore.

It has also been brought to my attention that having a preterm baby is one thing, but trying to care for kids and keep them alive is another. My therapist thinks I'm working myself into the ground due to my subconscious feeling of loss and fear that something will happen to Anson and Arisa. Maybe I am, and maybe I'm not. But I know I am raising my kids the best way I know how to.

At low moments, I feel like so much time, effort, emotion, money, work, and even my body have been given up for this goal of having a family. It's hard to have wanted kids so badly and then to some days feel like, *Why did I do this*? Do I regret it? NO WAY. Never. Our children are the best little things that have ever happened to me. But the picture of motherhood isn't painted realistically, and I think it's important to be honest.

As Mom, I wear all the hats. I'm chef, cleaner, chauffeur, disciplinarian, routine-maker, enforcer, and more. When Uche gets home, he jumps in and helps, but he will be the first to admit that he is able to take a break when he is at work. Uche has not lost himself. He can easily drop what he's doing to prioritize himself. Uche also recognizes that not much has changed for him other than we now have two beings to love and care for. He still goes to work. He still has his regular schedule. He still meets his buddies at the pub. I know that it is temporary. Once the kids are a little older and able to do more for themselves, I feel I will gain back more of myself.

When our babies were really little, everything felt very serious and regimented. It's a lot of responsibility. I was trying to figure out the needs and wants of our babies and trying to distinguish my own needs and wants. And now that they're a bit older and we're not taking things so seriously, it has been a lot of fun. Even now, with Arisa three and Anson eight, I'm starting to feel more like myself.

I now have a whole morning routine where I promise I won't do anything for anyone until I do these things for myself first: I wake up. I do not check my phone. I wash my face and get dressed (or not—depends on my mood, since we are at home). I started using essential oils, so I fill the diffuser, work out, and then make myself hot lemon water. Anson is online learning at the moment, and during his first class, I'm doing yoga. It sets the tone for the day and fills my cup a bit. The kids know that once

I'm done with yoga, "Mommy's ready." Sometimes the kids will join my yoga practice, and it's incredible to watch them move their bodies, learn new poses, and connect to their spirit. I've seen them implement some of the breathing techniques I do at random times in their day. They are sponges soaking everything in.

Writing this book has also been a part of finding Rena again and doing something for myself. It's all a process. I can start to feel Rena coming back more and more every day. There have been days within the past month where Uche has hugged me and said, "You're finally coming back to me."

Uche and Anson have their daily routines, too. Anson is an early riser, so he gets up on his own and hangs out with Uche in the office while Uche is working. If he is up before Uche, he will watch TV on his own. The morning is their "bro time," as they like to call it. Uche gets breakfast ready for the kids most days and after they are off to school, Uche will head back to the office for work.

Uche is the most hands-on, loving, patient, helpful, and entertaining father. He comes out of the office throughout the day just to check on everyone and make sure we are all happy. He doesn't mind when the kids barge into the office just to say "hi." He loves our family and the kids bring him so much joy.

The Joys of Motherhood

As a mother, I give a lot—but I will say that giving yields returns. It's amazing to see these little beings grow and understand the world around them with each passing day. For example, the other day, Arisa was going to eat something she shouldn't have. This girl puts everything in her mouth! Anson went over before I could say, "Arisa, we can't do that," and he calmly talked to her and was able to show her a different way. It was heartening.

When you're a parent, every milestone your child goes through is a huge deal. I have documented everything from first smiles, first laughs, first rolls, first crawls, and first time walking for both children. I am fortunate to have been present for all of those things for both kids. Seeing our kids go through stages brings us overwhelming joy. As they grow, we start to see their little personalities shining through and we help them foster their own interests and goals. Seeing excitement through our kids' eyes is such a gift.

I also realize things about myself I didn't know before. I didn't know I could love so deeply. Both kids have taught me patience I never knew I had. They taught me that my way of doing things is not the only way; we are all separate people with different needs and different wants and what works for one doesn't always work for the other. They've taught me unconditional love. They always push me to be my best. And they are always listening even when I don't think they are, so I'm constantly making sure I am modeling the behavior that I want them to see (as well as trying to say the F-word less often).

Their innocence keeps me grounded. A big thing for our family specifically is we love singing in the car. When they were toddlers, it was funny to hear them sing songs that toddlers wouldn't normally sing. When Anson was younger, he used to sing "No limits" by Usher, but it would come out as, "no wimits." One day we were driving, and he said, "Mom, I want you to call Usher." I said, "I don't have Usher's number, baby. But if I did, I would absolutely call him." He started full-on crying because I wouldn't call Usher for him. It's sweet to see how their minds work.

I have learned that it's the little things that make us smile. The belly laughs of children are the absolute, most infectious, loving, amazing sound ever. It's impossible not to join in. Uche and I are constantly watching the kids play and interact with each other, whether they're tickling or wrestling, or chasing each other. We've started playing Monopoly and Scrabble together. We do more board games now that Anson is able to read and participate in ways that he hasn't been able to before.

We do family sleepover nights where we will set up foamies in our room and the kids will sleep with us. Lately, it's turned into setting a tent up in the backyard with the boys going outside and the girls sleeping inside in the king bed. (I think we won there.) We have started doing family movie nights every Friday as a way to end the week. We set up a splat mat on the floor like a picnic, and the kids get to sit and eat while sitting on their marshmallow chairs. It's a time where I let go of rules and let them pick whatever snack they want. The pure, true, joy and smiles on their faces warm my body.

Kid snuggles are the absolute best. Arisa and I snuggle every day, especially while watching movies. She's my daytime snuggler. With Anson, we usually snuggle after our bedtime routine. I'll lay down with him for a bit and we will have our best conversations then, when it's quiet and just the two of us. Anson also opens up to Uche a lot in that setting.

When the kids come up to us and hug us for no reason, it is a body rush of pure warmth and joy. It solidifies for me that what we are doing is working. There are no manuals for raising children and what I do versus what my sister does versus what my friend does could be very different, so to see my kids happy and thriving, makes me feel like we are on the right track. When I get a hug or an "I love you" that's not prompted, I know that life is good.

There are some days when the kids will be outside and all I hear is laughter. I just watch them through the window and think, "There are my little miracles and they are such a joy," or, "Listen to their laughter." One time, I was watching them with Uche in complete amazement, pride, and joy and said, "Look at our family."

And he said, "I know. We did it. Look how cute our kids are."

I'm like, *I know*. "I'm so happy this is our life."

Conclusion

To all the mothers and fathers out there experiencing a journey of infertility, here is my perspective (rather than "advice"—advice is a tricky word because it's such an individual journey).

I am not going to tell you to relax—when I was going through infertility, I hated that word. When people told me to relax, I would bristle. However, being on the other side now, having gone through a miracle conception and birth, the truest point in my journey was when I was able to let go and accept my situation, and truly believe that whatever will be is what will be. I think what may have been more beneficial for me to hear than being told to relax, was being told to try and find balance.

I became so laser-focused on what I wanted that it encompassed my whole life: body, mind, and soul. Trying to get pregnant became a full-time job, in terms of going to appointments, giving myself injections, and having to schedule sex around a particular day and time. It was constant. If you can genuinely give your body over to it—but keep your mind and soul in a very comforting place—it's beneficial both for getting pregnant, but also for your peace of mind. I started saying, "It's off my plate," and tried not to think about it so much.

Once I let go of my rigid control, we were pregnant within two months, without even trying. The body is a very powerful thing. What I'm learning now is how much the psychological impacts the physical. I understand that better now than before. Before, I was almost militant about what I needed to do. *This is what I want, I'm going to do it and nothing's going to stop me.* If you had asked me back then, I would never have said I was stressed. Looking back, of course, I was. My job as a dental hygienist was affecting my body physically. Spending my day seated and hunched over patients was causing pain throughout my back. At that point, I was seeing a massage therapist every two weeks and getting acupuncture, physiotherapy, and seeing a chiropractor all at once just to maintain my shoulder and neck. I don't know if that had anything to do with it, but stress is stress, no matter how it comes.

At the time, I was looking at stress as a cataclysmic event of some kind, which I didn't feel, but stress comes in all forms, shapes, and sizes and is different for different people. Now I understand that stress is defined as the degree to which one feels overwhelmed or unable to cope as a result of pressures that are unmanageable. I also realized after the fact that there is more than one kind of stress. Columbia River Mental Health Services outlines three main different kinds of stress—acute stress, episodic acute stress, and chronic stress—each with its own characteristics, symptoms, duration, and treatment approaches.

If you can let go of the process a little bit and not be so rigid about it, it will help. Take time out for your body, nourish it, make sure you are in a state that promotes relaxation and comfort. Trust your body, trust the process, and try not to get wound up in it like I did, and it may go a bit smoother.

Now, when you're in it, of course, that's way easier said than done. The process is so clinical, the stakes are high, it's expensive, and everything is on a rigid schedule. You are told when to take medication, when to book your appointments, what to eat, and when to have sex. Everything is so regimented that it's hard to "relax." Find whatever can help you move away from all that intensity. Even though you're in it, detach a bit from it. Keep the focus and keep your eye on the prize—don't give up on your dream, but let go of your need to control it a little bit.

Also, trust your instincts. When we went to that first clinic, as soon as we walked in, both my husband and I felt icky. Check out your different options, if you have them. Once we found the second clinic, our experience, our vibe, our opinions, our comfort, our emotions—everything shifted.

If you've gone through a miscarriage or experienced another loss, you know that it is an intense and often lonely struggle. Because no one talks about it, it may feel like no one understands. Do what you need to do to get through it. In a moment like this, there is no judgment. And anyone who does judge, peace out. There is no right answer for how someone should handle a situation like this; we just need to get through it, *however we can.*

I saw a Reiki healer and a bunch of unprocessed grief and emotions came up during our session. "Your grief hasn't been dealt with properly," she said. Even today, whenever I talk about the loss of Ashtyn, I still shake. I still sweat. I still cry. I put that experience in a place where I can manage my day and it doesn't paralyze me, but it hasn't gone away. However, both Uche and I have found ways to honor her life and do our best to heal.

On Ashtyn's birthday, we light a candle. And we participate in Infant Loss Awareness month, a worldwide event where anyone and everyone lights a candle in their time zone on October 15 at 7 p.m. to commemorate their angel babies. Every year, we light Ashtyn's candle and another candle for our friend's baby, Jackson.

* * *

Faith played a role in our journey as well. I am proud to be Jewish, although I do not consider myself very religious. It's important to me to raise our children with faith and knowledge about Judaism. When we told Anson that I was pregnant with Arisa, he got super excited, jumped up and down, smiled and said, "It works."

"What worked?"

"I had prayed to God to ask for a baby and now we have a baby." To this day, my son says that the reason Arisa ended up in my belly is that he prayed to God.

An interesting thing to note is that I wasn't as faith-based until after Arisa was born because that's when I truly started believing that things happen for a reason. There is a higher power. Miracles do happen. Trust the process. These are all things that Arisa brought with her. I had been far too concerned with being in control at the beginning of our journey.

My wish for you is, wherever you are on your journey, that you find peace with where you are and with where you end up.

Husband's Perspective: Uche

At times, I feel like that process is over and everything's fine. But this morning, for example, I was getting the kids ready to go to the park, and Anson and Arisa were chatting away, and all I could think was, *Ashtyn should be with us.* They both know about Ashtyn now, so they'll talk about her. Arisa is learning her letters at the moment, so she will point out when she sees a letter she recognizes. "There's an A here." And Anson will say, "Oh yeah, Anson, Ashtyn, and Arisa." And Arisa will say, "Oh yeah, the three of us." And that brings back the emotions.

Every time I think we are past all of that, it comes back. We have pictures in our house symbolizing Ashtyn's memory. Our symbol for Ashtyn is a purple Hawaiian flower, and we have purple flowers at our front door to remember Ashtyn. She is always with us. We are not trying to forget that Ashtyn was here. We embrace that now. We are going forward, knowing that this is part of our story that's never going to disappear.

What I'd like to share with readers, especially with the men, is that your wife or partner might be experiencing different emotions, regardless of how you feel about it. To keep everything moving in a positive direction, I had to let go of judgment. It would be easy for a partner to say, "Hey, this happened six months ago. Come on, get back on the horse." Having that kind of attitude and judging your partner will not help.

Whatever Rena needed or wanted to do to cope is what we were going to do. She went through so much; she needed that kind of support. It wasn't up to me to decide whether she was worthy of the support or if she actually needed it. You don't need to think about whether she needs it or not. You just need to be there and support her, however long it takes. Maybe space alone is what she needs. Listen to her cues. If she needs to be around other people, then try to make suggestions, but don't force it.

When we started down this path, I often said to Rena, "Maybe part of the reason why we're not getting pregnant is stress." I could feel how stressed she was over the whole idea of getting pregnant. She had the idea in her mind that you have a kid and then you have another, two years apart. That's the perfect timing, right? So, she had all of these preconceived notions, schedules, and ideals, which weighed on all of us. Not just her, but all of us. She was also working at the time and her body was under a lot of physical stress. She has repetitive strain injuries in her arm and a lot of neck and back issues.

When we were going through this whole fertility journey, when we had Anson and were down to the last embryo and had a surrogate, there was no pressure on her whatsoever. That's when Arisa came. For me, looking back with 20/20 hindsight, I do believe that our complications were ultimately due to stress. The pressures of trying to have this perfect family with kids two years apart, all of these things that we built up and put on ourselves, the pressure and the timelines, and the work schedules, stressed us out. But when we were able to say, "Okay, we're good with whatever happens in the next few months," we were able to have a child naturally.

Acknowledgments

First and foremost, thank you Anson for making me a mom, and teaching me unconditional love. Thank you, Arisa, for making me believe in miracles. And thank you Ashtyn, for showing me the strength I didn't know I had.

Uche, you are my rock. Thank you for always standing by me through the craziness. I know our experience was a roller coaster that consumed our whole marriage. Toward the end of this journey, it was my need that drove this process forward, and I really respect you for allowing it to continue for so long. I don't think I tell you enough: I love you. Plus, you are the best dad!

Mom, thank you for helping us navigate every step of our fertility journey; for instantly scooping me up and holding me through every loss; for helping me understand every physical symptom I had pre- and post-partum; for caring for me and my family when I couldn't; and for being the best Nana. Dad, thank you for always being the calm and logical one; for your constant advice about navigating through life; for your trust;

and for all our daddy-daughter talks. These talks mean the world to me. Anson and Arisa are so lucky you're their Papa.

To Jana and Matt, for opening up your house to us, supporting us during treatments and during loss, going to appointments with me, helping me with medications, and providing endless playtime with Hunter and Hayden to keep us smiling through it all.

Melissa, thank you for selflessly offering your own body to help us complete our journey, and for being there every step of the way. I firmly believe you are the reason we got pregnant naturally. Thank you for taking the pressure off. Forever connected.

To Carla, for showing up and guiding me in my darkest time. Even when you said you didn't know how, you knew how. Thank you for always listening and allowing space for every single emotion I had without judgment; for helping me with Anson when I couldn't; for being our family.

To Kylie, for crying with me after I delivered Ashtyn and for picking me up when I thought I couldn't move on. You were the first person I talked to when we got back from the hospital. Even though we're far away, our hearts are always close together.

Thank you, Carly and Brandon, for always knowing what to say, when to say it, how to say it, and for never letting our experience dim your shine.

Thank you, Adele, for your e-mails and texts, endless thoughtful words, and medical expertise. You talk me through my toughest moments.

To Terry and David, for completely taking us under your wing when we moved to Houston and instantly making us part of your family. Thank you for always including us and treating us as members of your own.

To Paul, Lee, Dawn, and Aric for opening up to us, guiding us, comforting us, and holding us through the deepest loss when you were going through it yourselves. Thank you for your endless love and support always.

To my crew, Jodi, Peri, Nikki, and Katy for centering me, grounding me, understanding me. Thank you for our annual girls' trips, for forever fun, for loving whole-heartedly through thick and through thin, and for always believing in me. Love you girls for life.

To Natalie, for allowing me to continue to harass you about stopping my labor, and for always trying to be by my side after loss—even when I wasn't receptive to it. Thank you for not giving up on me.

Thank you, Erin, for giving me my first-ever injection because I couldn't do it myself. You rocked it!

To Dr. Faghih for truly making this experience more comfortable. Your genuine approach to care supported us when we needed it the most. Thanks for helping us start our family, you will always be one of our favorites.

Dr. Cowan, thank you for keeping your promise and getting my miracle pregnancy to term. You are a fabulous doctor and played a pivotal role in completing our family. Forever grateful for you.

ABOUT THE

Author

Rena Ejiogu traveled the infertility gauntlet from 2009 to 2017. When trying naturally didn't work, Rena and her husband, Uche, tried everything from Clomid to intrauterine insemination (IUI) to in vitro fertilization (IVF) to surrogacy. Throughout the process, Rena experienced the heartbreak of seven miscarriages including

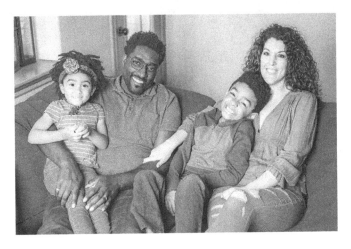

one preterm birth. Today, Rena is the proud mom of two beautiful children and has found strength through sharing her journey with other women and couples struggling with infertility.

Rena is available for speaking engagements. Please e-mail **renaejiogu@gmail.com** for more information.

Appendix

Cost of Fertility Treatments

Costs of fertility treatments vary significantly between the United States and Canada, but when we went through our fertility treatments, nothing was covered under any sort of healthcare. They have since made changes in Canada. I know there are now portions that are covered in Ontario, but when we were going through it, all the treatments were out of pocket.

Please note prices depicted in this book are an estimate and based on the time of treatment. Prices have increased over the years, and procedure costs differ between clinics and patients.

Medications were mostly covered by our healthcare, so we only had to pay a portion of my medications. In Calgary, at the time I did the IUIs, they were $325 a pop, and I did three rounds. So, we spent $975 on IUIs alone. They may cost considerably more now.

Our IVF costs in Ontario were $15,664.15, which doesn't include any medication expenses, plane tickets, hotel rooms, or time off work.

The total bill for Regional Fertility Clinic in Calgary was $9,825, which doesn't include any annual administration fee, embryo freezing, annual embryo storage, any medication expense, or time off work.

It's also worth mentioning that for frozen embryos, there is a storage fee. We had frozen embryos left after both rounds of IVF, which we paid a yearly fee to have stored. We had five left at ONE Fertility after the first round (with which I was implanted), and the last two that the surrogate used. It wasn't until we decided to go the surrogate route that we paid attention to those embryos. Embryo storage at the Ontario clinic was $353.98 for the year. We had to pay that three times. In total, we paid over a thousand dollars to store embryos at the Ontario clinic. The fee at the Calgary clinic was similar, around $400 for the year. We also paid a company to transport our embryos from Calgary to Burlington, which was close to another $1,000.

There is also a fee for what is called "assisted hatching," which is the thawing process, that was $400 at the Ontario clinic. There's a fee for every little step. It adds up. Any little added expense felt opportunistic. *Of course, there's a fee.*

For surrogacy, we offered to pay all the attorney's fees. Our lawyer fee for our contract with Melissa was $4,500. We also covered things like gas money, wages for time she had to take off work, any prescriptions, etc.

COST OF FERTILITY TREATMENTS

		ONE FERTILITY	REGIONAL FERTILITY PROGRAM
1	Annual Admin Fee	$253	$300
2	IUI	-	$325/round x 3= $975
3	IVF	$7200	$7700
4	ICSI	$1500	$1600
5	Sperm Wash	$550	?
6	Embryo Freezing	$850	$1050
7	Assisted Hatching	$400	$500
8	Embryo Thawing & Transfer	$1,800 x2 = $3600	-
9	Annual Embryo Storage	$354 x 3 = $1,062	$396
10	Medications	?	Range $3,000 - $8,000

ADDITIONAL FEES

Embryo Transfer Calgary → Burlington	$842
Surrogate Lawyer Fees	$3000 (ours) $1,500 (surrogate) =
	$4500

TOTAL: ≈ $41, 275 *

* Total fee does not include taxes
* Plane tickets, hotel rooms, time off work to be factored in to total cost as well.

Fertility can be expensive depending on the route you go. We were fortunate to be able to put any bonus that Uche received from work towards fertility, and we were very fortunate that my parents offered to pitch in with our second round of IVF. We were in a good position, which I do not take for granted. But I can tell you, I would have found a way no matter what. That's how badly I wanted it and how important it was to me. Can you put a price on having a family? Ours was in the $50,000-$80,000 range (and these are outdated rates). When associated costs are added in—plane tickets, room and board, missed pay from being absent from work, etc., it was probably closer to $100,000.

9 781636 498850